# Chronic Illness:

## Learning to live behind my smile

Copyright @2019 Jane L Edwards

ISBN 9781075727863

All rights reserved.

A very big thank you to my wonderful family for putting up with me for the last decade, it has been a tough journey, and I couldn't have survived it without your love and support.

Special thank you to S, C and C for living this challenge every day with me, I know I can be a nightmare.

Thank you to Alex, Jane and Neil for their voluntary editorial role, I really appreciate the time and effort you put in to try and improve my ramblings.

And finally thank you to all my friends and family for love and support, even when I cannot quite face the world.

Jx

Quick legal comment, this book is my journey, none of the statements is personal advice for you, if you need personalised help, please speak with your doctor.

# Contents

| | |
|---|---|
| Why should you read this book? | 5 |
| What is a Chronic Illness? | 7 |
| Hello, this is me | 8 |
| My stages | 15 |
| Talking about 'it.' | 47 |
| Pacman | 56 |
| Who is your battle with? | 62 |
| Who to trust with your health? | 75 |
| Cheese sandwich again? | 86 |
| Remission, relapse are just words | 93 |
| Inspiring? Me? | 101 |
| Learning to trust yourself | 108 |
| Everybody has their own battles | 122 |
| Fragility | 127 |
| Invisible illness | 131 |
| My personal thoughts on … | 139 |
| Changes we can make from today; master of my fate. | 161 |
| Final word | 163 |
| Reference website | 164 |
| About the Author: Jane L Edwards | 166 |

## Why should you read this book?

The problem with a long-term chronic illness is that it isn't a quick fight, taking a few drugs and having a couple of weeks in bed will not cure it. It isn't ever an out and out win, you never beat the illness forever. It is a long-term war, some battles you lose and some you win: It is an on-going campaign. It is a chronic illness, after all.

In the end, the struggle is about getting to a place where you can live together, the illness and you, and trying to make the most of the environment you share, an attempt to make it a positive life.

This book is a collection of experiences I have faced living with a chronic illness, experiences I am still learning from and having to deal with every day. It is like living in no man's land, somewhere between feeling ill and feeling healthy, but not really being healthy or ill. I hope, by sharing my experience, I can help you with your journey, dealing with your chronic illness or give you some tools to help you make some sense of living with a chronic condition.

I need to tell you something up front: I don't have a magic solution to deal with chronic illness. I cannot sell you a magic pill or a special diet to make all this better for you and I don't have one piece of mind-blowing advice (that I obviously trademark and make a fortune); I can't give you tricks that will cure everything and make you look like a swimwear model.

The book is an honest representation of my battle, and some of the small changes I have made that have added up to some significant improvements in my life. The book shares lessons I have learned on my tough journey of six years trying to get back to a 'normal life' with a rare illness. It contains ideas on how to take control of your life, where to find help and what to do if the people who should be helping you don't live up to your expectations.

- Read this if you want some truthful advice from somebody who is a few years ahead of you on the journey you may be about to face. The book contains the information I wish I had been given in the first stages of my illness, which could have made my journey a lot easier from the very start. I did not receive any useful information about what to expect and how to cope with these vast changes, so I hope a little information will help you along your journey.

- Do not read this if you want a magic trick that may cost you a lot of money and has no basis in science or research. Magic cures don't exist, but if you want to read how sometimes they can appear too, read about the power of the placebo effect.[1]

Chronic illnesses are challenging to deal with, as there is no end to the battle in sight, and they are with you for life. Therefore, to get the most from your life you must learn to live with the illness and all the quirks it brings to your life. Each illness is different, and each illness can affect people in different ways.

**The book is not about your illness or mine, but about how to get the best from your situation and how to negotiate the health system; about small changes that can help you to remain positive and wake up each morning with enough fight in your belly to face the day.**

---

[1] http://www.nhs.uk/Livewell/complementary-alternative-medicine/Pages/placebo-effect.aspx

## What is a Chronic Illness?

The World Health Organization (WHO) say that chronic conditions require:

> "on-going management over a period of years or decades" and cover a wide range of health problems that go beyond the conventional definition of chronic illness, such as heart illness, diabetes and asthma. They include some communicable illnesses, such as the human immunodeficiency virus and the acquired immunodeficiency syndrome (HIV/AIDS), transformed by advances in medical science from rapidly progressive fatal conditions into controllable health problems, allowing those affected to live with them for many years. They also extend to certain mental disorders such as depression and schizophrenia, to defined disabilities and impairments not defined as illnesses, such as blindness and musculoskeletal disorders (WHO 2002), and to cancer, the subject of a separate volume published by the European Observatory (Coleman et al. 2008)." [2]

From this passage, I take a chronic illness to be any illness which you need to live with for years. As treatments for initial illnesses improve, more of us will be living with long-term conditions that change our everyday life without us ever receiving a complete 'cure'. Some illnesses will have minimal effects; others will drastically change your life and that of your family and friends. Chronic illnesses can leave you feeling more vulnerable and uncertain about the future, and most will need to be managed daily to cope effectively with the impact they bring to your life.

---

[2] http://www.euro.who.int/__data/assets/pdf_file/0006/96468/E91878.pdf

## Hello, this is me

I finally have accepted my illness is permanent, I think. It will never go away. There is no magic pill I can take to cure everything. Short of some amazing medical breakthrough, I must face reality and live with this illness for the rest of my life.

It has taken me years to realise this permanence. Most of my friends and family understood the permanence of the illness a long time ago, but I'm stubborn and thought, "Hey! I can beat this, if I only eat well and push myself to get healthier and fitter, and if I manage to sleep well, and I take vitamins and …". Six years later it has sunk in: I'm living with this illness forever. But somehow the realisation has given me freedom. A freedom I have been missing for those six years. Freedom to decide how to live with it, and freedom to reconsider all my long-held pre-conceptions of what my life would be like at 40 years' old. A chance to look at life differently and a chance to decide what is really important. Don't worry, I won't be suggesting that you must change everything in your life and run off and be a Nun or a Monk. I will share some of the changes I have made and some of the lessons I have learnt along the journey.

My 'epiphany' has taken a while. When I first became ill, I thought it would be like a Hollywood movie where within two hours you get ill, you fight hard, you realise who loves you, and you win the battle. You reassess your life and at the end of the movie you are happier than before you got ill; you have realised what really matters and your hair and makeup are perfect throughout or for guys you still have your 6 pack and a fabulous suntan. A wonderful fairy-tale.

I thought being stuck with this meant I had to come out of it with some major realisation or significant life-changing actions. I haven't.

**I should really have been concentrating all my efforts and energies on getting stronger and healthier, rather than on some fake fantasy about changing the world**

because of what I'll overcome in my personal life. I felt like the only one in the word dealing with a major challenge.

I did not write this book to motivate you to climb a mountain or start a multimillion-pound charity (I don't know how to do either of these things). I wrote the book with the idea of giving you suggestions of things I wish people had told me at the time of my diagnosis. I cannot give you medical answers to your condition or mine, but I will help with some of the things you may face while coming to terms with a chronic illness and getting back to a life that you can be happy living. I have no medical qualifications (but, if you need this support, you should seek expert advice from people who know your full medical history). I do hope that I can help you make the most of what you have, and I bet that when you look at the world around you, you will have many good things very close to you. Sometimes we just cannot see them and need a kind reminder of where to look for the good things in our life.

I do make light of some aspects of my experience. I am not misunderstanding the seriousness of things, but it is the easiest way I have found to deal with my condition. People say I am always so positive and cheerful no matter what is thrown at me; this could not be further from the truth – just ask my husband! I hide it well, and I have learnt to present a positive face in public. But there are both good and bad aspects of putting on a brave face.

Not all the material will be relevant to everybody who reads it. I talk a little about rare conditions, which will not be relevant to everybody but may give those without a rare illness a few useful ideas.

Shall we start with the first question most people ask when diagnosed with any life-changing condition?

**WHY ME?**

It is a natural question. We immediately think "Why Me?" because we feel the world is not being fair to us. But are we really that unlucky? I knew a nurse a few years ago who had frequent contact with cancer patients, and the most common question she ever had was, Why Me?

Her comment to me was, respectfully, **"Why NOT you?"** Sounds cruel? She really didn't mean it nastily, and when you look at the facts, you can start to understand her twist on the question.

The statistics are astounding (all references taken in July 2016):

- There were around 352,000 new cases of cancer in the UK in 2013, that's 960 cases diagnosed every day.[3] Half (50%) of people diagnosed with cancer in England and Wales survive their illness for ten years or more (2010-11).[4]

- Since 1996 the number of people diagnosed with diabetes in the UK has more than doubled, from 1.4 million to almost 3.5 million.[5]

- 7.3 million people in England have sought treatment for osteoarthritis. This represents 33% of the population over 45.[6]

- One in six people aged 80 and over have dementia. 60,000 deaths a year are directly attributable to dementia.[7]

- In the UK 600,000, or one in every 103, people have epilepsy.[8]

---

[3] http://www.cancerresearchuk.org/health-professional/cancer-statistics/incidence

[4] http://www.cancerresearchuk.org/health-professional/cancer-statistics

[5] https://www.diabetes.org.uk/About_us/What-we-say/Statistics/

[6] http://www.arthritisresearchuk.org/arthritis-information/data-and-statistics/data-by-condition/osteoarthritis.aspx

[7] https://www.alzheimers.org.uk/statistics

[8] https://www.epilepsy.org.uk/press/facts

- A rare illness at some point in their lives will affect 1 in 17 people or 7% of the population.[9]

When I look at these figures, I agree that the question shifts to '**why not me?**' Each of us has a high chance of contracting an illness we must live with for the rest of our lives; some may be easier to handle than others. Some people may be better at managing what is thrown at them than others. Some of us have high pain thresholds and some, like me, are complete wimps about pain.

We all need to find our own way to cope. Some try to be heroes and show others what humans are capable of, while some soldier on silently without telling anybody. **It is your decision about how to react; what works for you, your personality, situation and illness. There is no correct reaction to dealing with a chronic illness diagnosis. One important action is to not compare your way of coping with the symptoms or drug side effects with anybody else's method of coping; they are personal, and this really is not a competition.**

Occasionally, when I really hate my illness, I think what it would be like to have some of the other illnesses in the world and how I would cope with those. Some seem more straightforward to understand, some seem scarier, but none of them seems to be much fun. Generally, I conclude that this thought process is a waste of time, and I should just get on with my current life.

Maybe, by looking at the question differently, it is easier to deal with. Perhaps we should ask ourselves a few other questions to help us put everything in perspective:

- Why not me?

- Which illness would I pick, if it were my choice?

- Could my illness make me mentally stronger?

- Will I learn more about myself from facing this illness?

[9] http://www.rareillness.org.uk/about-rare-illnesses.htm

- Also, my personal favourite question ... **How can I NOT let it beat me?**

How can I NOT let it beat me? This is where I have chosen to focus my energies: a positive question about what I can do with the cards dealt to me.

I remember the consultant sitting at the end of my hospital bed, after two weeks of waiting for answers, explaining to me what my biopsy had found and trying to describe my illness. The conversation took about five minutes, then he went straight onto the drugs I would need and the side effects, including increased risk to what seemed like every illness possible plus the dreaded steroid weight gain and moon face. There was no discussion around how to cope mentally with this news, or how to adapt physically to the changes this would bring to my life after the first month. No specialist nurse came to see me. I received a BIG bag of drugs and a discharge letter, and I went home and cried for a long time.

A little while later I woke up and declared I could fight this and win. Little did I really understand my challenge, but I would soon start to realise the implications of this life change.

Some chronic illnesses have great marketing and PR teams who fight for fundraising. They bring in sponsorship and fund specialist nurses who can care and support you through the journey, which is excellent for those patients who are supported by these teams. However, many illnesses don't have this resource or support, mine included. It can lead to a feeling that healthcare is not equally distributed, and this can build a little resentment. Unfortunately, it did for me. I understand that it is often because people can understand something like breast cancer, and this makes it easier to understand, which allows the knowledge to be shared efficiently. When I was diagnosed, some of my friends said to me *'thank god it isn't cancer'*. It made me feel that everybody believed that, because I wasn't diagnosed with cancer, I wasn't really in any danger from my illness.

Some of the medical fundraising and PR teams have done a fantastic job and have very cleverly brought in enormous amounts of money for research. This will help everybody in the UK (and I congratulate all involved for fighting for their cause). However, well-known diseases are not the only ones that can destroy lives. Shortly after my diagnosis, a news story broke where Pancreatic Cancer Action used the words, 'I wish I had Breast Cancer'; it caused shock and outrage[10]. I can really understand both sides, but I am not sure the UK press really tried to put forward both sides of the story. I have referenced an article published after the beautiful girl in the campaign, Kerry Harvey, had died. I cannot imagine the strength it took Kerry to front this campaign.

One of the last things Kerry said on record was:

> "Hopefully, the campaign will lead to more money being spent on research into pancreatic cancer. It won't help me, but I hope it will mean others will have a better chance than I have."

I understand what the campaign was trying to tell people: there are many illnesses in the world, some understood more than others and some better funded than others, but it doesn't seem fair that a person's chance of survival depends on how good the fundraising team of a charity performs. It is not about jealousy or hatred; it is about distributing funding to support all those struggling with an illness. We have a long way to go before things are equal and fair in healthcare. I think Kerry was amazingly brave and I hope her family can take courage from the knowledge that she made a difference. **The fundamental fact is that we should not decide to fund healthcare research or treatment by the size and capability of the charities that promote them.**

One more introductory comment: I would like to warn you that I love a good cliché. I think cliches are great; they become clichés because they originate from the truth. I will use some in the book. I think we sometimes need them for motivation and inspiration, but I promise not to overload you with them.

Nevertheless, I always have in my head the saying:

**What doesn't kill you makes you stronger.**

(However, I will add the warning, that some days you may feel crap and strong may be the last word you would use to describe how you feel!)

[10] http://www.huffingtonpost.co.uk/2014/02/25/kerry-harvey-pancreatic-cancer-dies_n_4853256.html

I hope you can come on this journey with me; I am still on my bumpy road as I write (so you may notice some moments when I am 'lower' than others). This is NOT a medical book or a self-help book; it is just my brain sharing things my family and I have learnt along the way, and I hope these can help you in your personal journey.

We might not have the same illness, or be the same age or sex, but we will face some of the same challenges, tests, giggles and frustrations. So, I say let us try to live life to the maximum with our chronic illness and see what benefits this change in our life could bring to us. Maybe your favourite question will become the same as mine:

### How can I NOT let this illness beat me?

About me? Well, I am a little over 40, married to a man who loves me dearly but thinks that discussing anything emotional is a waste of energy. We have two beautiful girls aged eight and thirteen. I work four days a week in technical marketing, but I am fortunate to have a fantastic employer who has allowed me to be flexible during my years of treatment (I cannot thank them enough). My children have contributed a lot to this book, because they are children and, as such, say things exactly as they are. Somehow most of their comments really make me giggle:

- Mum, you look like a ghost today!
- When will that extra tummy be gone, mummy?
- But mummy it's just not fair we are not well either (as a drop of snot dribbles from her nose).

Reality is never far away with children, but that is good. It helps you to keep fighting and really understand that you cannot let anything beat you, because you need to keep listening to the honest statements made by those you share your life with. Love you S, C and C xxx.

## My stages

Everything is always easier to deal with if broken into small sections, like cooking, running or origami. We are currently enjoying making a 'sitting fox' for homework and have got slightly obsessed with following the steps to make it. If you fancy a few fun hours, search the internet for 'origami fox sitting'. When I look back, I find it much easier to describe the sequence of events of my illness by breaking it into stages. You will follow a different path, or maybe skip steps or have additional challenges along the way. Again, please remember I am not offering medical advice here; just sharing some of the realistic experiences I faced, in the hope that it might make life a little easier for you as you face your upcoming challenges.

### Pre-illness

I was blindly ambitious, so desperate to prove I could do anything and everything. The ignorance of youth maybe, but I worked hard, and I committed fully to my job. I travelled all over the world for meetings, I met the most amazing people, and I stayed in beautiful five-star hotels, continually working. My husband did the same. We thought we had a great life, and in a way we did. I wouldn't change any of it, but I also wouldn't go back there now. After a couple of months of being married, I fell pregnant with my first baby girl.

The pregnancy was good, I felt happy, and I carried on working long hours, right up to the end. At this point, I had a great Italian boss who was family orientated and supported me in a kind manner, and often told me how much the birth would hurt as this made him laugh wildly with sarcasm.

All was good.

At least I pretended all was good. I was tired and had been for many years. I had very little sex drive or time for fun, other than going for a few beers down the pub. Putting it down to a full-on job, I ignored the nagging feeling that something was not quite right. Throughout my journey, and subsequently writing about my experience, I have learnt that I am very skilled at pretending all is good and showing a 'rose tinted' version of myself to everybody. One of my favourite songs is Billy Joel's 'The Stranger' and, looking back, I hid a large part of me behind a happy smiling face. The song talks about a face that you hide and only show when everybody has gone.

I did not hide my feelings maliciously or in any kind of strategic manner. I am not some horrible scheming person pretending to be somebody else; it is merely my way of coping. I still do it now. If I smile and act as though all is right in the world, maybe, just maybe, it will be. **This strategy works until you realise nobody can help you if you continuously pretend all is right in the world. They can only help when you show the less than perfect side of you.** I still haven't worked out how to do this entirely; there is always a little bit left hidden from public view.

My unborn daughter didn't want to leave the comfort of my huge belly. So at twelve days overdue, chemical measures were started to get her out (please don't worry, I am not going into any graphic details here). Eventually, she arrives 15 days late. I lost consciousness and significant amounts of blood. I felt I had failed her by not being there right when she needed me. Logically, I know this is nonsense, but emotionally, I felt exhausted and vulnerable. However, after several blood transfusions, I started to feel brighter and more capable.

I wasn't a natural mother and struggled with the massive change in our lives and the routine it brought me. I loved my little family with everything I had, but I really did struggle in those first months, or maybe even years. I thought it would get easier and as one midwife said, 'Alpha women always struggle'. What she meant, in a kind way, was that women who had been successful in their chosen career really struggled when they became Mums. What I heard was that it was my fault. They are suddenly nowhere near experts, bombarded with often contradictory advice or comments on what they should be doing. I am not sure the midwife's comments helped at the time, but they have helped me when I look back on how difficult it was for our family and me.

Eventually, I did start to admit something wasn't quite right physically. At first, I thought it was from the trauma of the birth, but my husband, in one of his more sensitive moments, pointed out it had been going on from before that. However, a few months after giving birth, I got back to a stage where I could hide my reality again from the world and carry on as though I was living the dream. Therefore, that is what I did, and still, I thought I did it perfectly and that nobody else had any idea of how I felt inside.

**Starting to realise I was ill**

I was not really fooling anybody close to me; they could all see the struggles I was going through. However, I am not an easy person to tell what to do; generally, I do not listen to people when they say I cannot do something. Instead of listening to the concerns, I go off trying to prove I can do anything (Yes, I agree, I am a real nightmare). One day, while visiting my Mother with my new-born baby, my wonderful friend (who also happens to be a GP) sat me down and clearly, in simple terms, told me that things were not normal and she was worried about my health and made me promise to go and talk to my GP.

When I got home, I went to see my GP, and he was brilliant, but at the time, I don't think I was completely honest about everything. Or maybe I just didn't know exactly how to explain my symptoms and feelings, but we concluded it was post-natal depression.

I accepted this diagnosis as I was so desperately in need of a solution that could get me back to enjoying life again.

As I said, he was a good GP, so off I went for some counselling, which brought up many things I didn't know were there. I respect people in my life too much to write about any of it here but, pointedly, the counselling didn't help me physically.

No physical improvement at all: None, Zip, Nada, Nothing, Zero, Zilch. I felt very disappointed; what was wrong with me?

Psychologically it helped me to realise important things, and I have revisited these over the last few years, but it did not solve my tiredness or inability to think straight, or the visual disturbances I would get.

I went onto anti-depressants tablets. I had never considered I would need such a thing and, if I am honest, I hated taking them with a passion. Of course, I never said that to anybody; I gave the line of, "if you broke your leg you would seek treatment, so what is the difference if your head needs treatment?" I still had a lot to learn about all types of illness at this point in the journey. The drugs helped me to think a little straighter, and the counselling helped me to understand my past a bit better, but I still didn't physically feel any improvement. I saw a Consultant who said the visual disturbances were probably a migraine. This confused me as I never had a headache, and they only happened when I was exhausted.

**However, if a consultant tells you something, then you tend to believe them they know what they are talking about, so I accepted the simple diagnosis.**

So now I had post-natal depression and migraines, I ignored both and carried on. Can you see the pattern here? In all honesty, I have only realised how dangerous this pattern of ignoring symptoms was once I started writing it all down. I couldn't understand what I was doing at all until I documented the journey on paper for this book.

I returned to work part-time, 3 days a week, with the idea of having a great work life balance. I felt guilty at work, and I often worked on my days at home. I was still just 'not quite right'. I used up all the energy I could muster on my child and work. Again, I must apologise to my husband for him coming at the end of the list; I am sorry.

I wanted to 'pull myself together', so I tried various routes to help myself:
- I went to the Gym;

- I went to see a nutritionist and did not really learn anything new, other than that fact that supplements are expensive;

- I went to see an acupuncturist and saw no change at all;

- I walked the dog.

I tried, and I tried, and I tried to feel ok, but none of these actions helped me at all. Then I got pneumonia. I was thirty-something years' old for God's sake, and you do not get pneumonia in your thirties; that is an old person's illness (again, I had a lot to learn). I gave in for a couple of weeks and rested, as much as you can with a young child.

I had been sent for a chest scan over Christmas, and the delays meant that it was weeks before I had the scan and got the results. The GP had told me that if I had been 70 and a smoker, he would have sworn it was cancer… this wasn't really what I wanted to hear.

Therefore, I fought back and worked through it. Looking back now, this evidence on the chest X-ray was probably down to my chronic illness, and it should have been picked up as something serious, but it was not.

Around the same time, I had a new boss at work. I knew the combination of being part-time, having a child that led to limited travel and now pneumonia was not a great career move in their eyes. I really was starting to feel the pressure from all sides. I returned to work before I was fit and healthy, but I felt I had no choice. With my big smile firmly drawn in place, nobody had a clue. Or so I thought. One lovely lady, who is still a special friend knew. She could see me struggle, she knew when my vision had gone, or when I couldn't walk up the stairs as my legs wouldn't get me up there with my laptop as it felt so bloody heavy and I couldn't breathe. I am grateful to her for being so lovely, and always will be, as I could not have survived those months without her support and kindness.

Then things seemed to pick up, I was pregnant, I so wanted another child, and now that was happening. It would all be all right.

**No longer able to hide everything.**

I have thought hard about whether I should include the next little bit in the book. Please be aware this is not the full story, with respect to my family.

We had a miscarriage, not in a very nice way, and then I lost my job.

My mask fell to the floor, and tears took over me for months. There are so many people who I am grateful to for sticking by me at this time; people who were close, and those who I hardly knew. I thank them with all my heart.

Understandably I thought that this was my rock bottom, and it was the lowest point for the next few years.

I got pregnant again and successfully had my beautiful second daughter four years after the first. Our family was complete, and I had not gone back to my career as I had decided to take a few years off to get healthy and enjoy being a Mum. I started running and through stubborn determination, completed a half-marathon (not very fast, but who cares). I went to spin classes and went back to the nutritionist; I was determined to get fit and healthy this time. I was desperate for something to work.

But I was not really feeling any fitter. At the end of the half-marathon, my husband and friend had laughed that my lips were blue; I had been plagued by cramp in my toes for the second half of the 13 miles. Of course, I ignored it. In my usual way of ignoring everything that was staring me in the face, I decided it was time to start looking to get back into employment. I think this is a typical story, **ignoring the minor symptoms and 'pushing through' thinking it is nothing and secretly hoping it will just go away. Please don't overlook the signs, go and get checked out if you have that little nagging voice in your head.**

After a few months of job hunting, I found a great job, mostly working from home, which allowed me to juggle family and work together perfectly. I started with my induction training with pure joy and excitement: several weeks in the office and childcare all planned; off I went to start my shiny new job.

I loved this job and still do, and I cannot pass on enough praise for my employer and my new boss for how they handled what was to come and continue for the next seven years. Thank you. I really do appreciate all your support and kindness. The training was perfect. It was so good to be in a company that valued quality above all else, where I had the chance to learn everyday … if only I could get rid of this tooth infection.

I apparently had a tooth infection. All the symptoms were there: pain, fever, not able to sleep despite going to bed at 7pm. I went to the dentist; he removed the troublesome wisdom teeth, all four of them. He removed all four, which seemed a little strange at the time. How could all four be infected at once? Two weeks later, nothing had changed. Three lots of antibiotics later and my dentist calmly says:

> 'It is not your teeth; you need to go and see your doctor; something is not quite right'.

I will not type the swear words I said, I was so frustrated to be slowed down by a simple tooth infection. Off I went back to the doctor with some more random, vague, minor, symptoms again… I had lost count how many times I had done the same routine over the last few years. **So many illnesses have the symptom of fatigue, or aching, just because we do not have obvious symptoms does not make them less real, my vague symptoms ended up being linked to a life-threatening disease. I just wish I had admitted the extent of how it was affecting my life earlier, many illnesses start slowly if in doubt, we should get checked out.**

However, this time, the blood tests did confirm something was wrong, but it was not clear what exactly it might be. The GP told me it was not anything to worry about, and it would not be anything serious. I carried on at work and taking care of the kids as usual, but I was a lot slower and covered in sweat most of the time. The GP referred me to a 'general hospital' consultant through my employer's private healthcare. I never got a chance to make it to the private doctors' appointment.

My appointment was booked for Monday morning. On the Thursday before, I took the kids to school. I felt terrible, and by the time I got back to the car, I was dripping with sweat and couldn't lift my head off the steering wheel; I felt exhausted. This had become a normal feeling, getting back into the car and collapsing forward for a few minutes to recover myself, but today was different. No recovery came this time. I sat there for maybe 15 minutes, utterly oblivious to anything around me. Finally, I made myself drive the mile and a half home. My clothes were wet through, and my face looked like I had run the full marathon. My legs were mush; I got through the front door and collapsed onto the bottom step. I grabbed a glass of water and went to walk up to my office on the third floor. I couldn't get up four steps. I stopped, and I sat down and did not move. I could not move.

**Finally, I realised this was serious and admitted the full extent of the symptoms to myself. My brain had just had a little epiphany and understood that it wasn't strong trying to carry on, it was just plain stupidity. The fact that I only stopped once I couldn't walk up four steps show how ridiculously I was behaving.**
**Starting diagnosis**

It had taken many years to get to this point, I'm not sure how many as I don't remember when it all started, but more than four. I could not ignore the symptoms anymore, so I called for an emergency appointment with the doctor. They could see me that afternoon, so without telling anybody what had happened, I carried on working that day, including an international phone conference that I conducted while lying down in my bed in flowery P-Js. I agree this was nuts!

At the doctors, there was an urgency now. I could barely stand and, after some initial heart monitoring and a phone call to the renal doctor at the nearby hospital, I was admitted as an emergency to the hospital that evening. I would like to tell you all about my complex emotions at this point, but I really did not have any; I was too exhausted to think of anything. I phoned my husband and told him he had to come home and take me to the hospital. I called my lovely Mother-in-law and asked her to come and look after the children. Then I packed, unemotionally and very-very slowly, mostly while sitting on the bed.

On the way to the hospital, I emailed my new boss and said I was being admitted to the hospital, but I would just work from the hospital. His reply was, kindly, don't dare work. For him and all my colleagues, this came entirely out of the blue as I hadn't mentioned anything to anybody about feeling ill. I had been at the company for six weeks, and people did not really know me so they could not see the difference in me from before the illness.

Now, I need a little rant here about how the healthcare system works in the UK. Yes, it is mostly incredible, and yes, it is free, if you ignore the National Insurance we pay, but it is NOT great when you go into an Accident and Emergency Department.

I had an admittance letter from my GP; I had approval for admittance to the hospital via a hospital consultant on the phone two hours before I arrived at the hospital. However, I waited for three and half-hours to see anybody. I sat slumped in the corner of the waiting room, unable to hold my head up, waiting. Surely, there is a better way to organise the A&E departments. I have watched the workings of many hospital departments over the years and have a few ideas on how these could improve, and it is not about throwing more money and resources at the problem.

When I eventually saw a doctor, he took so many samples of blood, blood cultures and one test that the nurse said she had never seen in her ten years in A&E; I wanted answers, but mostly I really wanted to go to sleep. It was now getting late in the evening, so I was admitted to the emergency short stay ward. I stayed in the hellhole for three nights, all through the weekend. I would like at this point to say this is when you see the worst of the UK population: so drunk they need admitting to the hospital, so desperate for a cigarette even though they have been told it will kill them that they sneak into the toilets to smoke. I was tired but felt too scared to sleep and no, I am not exaggerating: drunks falling, shouting, hitting, walking into the wrong beds, arguing and crying. I am tough, but I needed out. The nurses really deserved a medal; personally, I would have left some of these patients to damage themselves if they had talked to me the way they spoke to those nurses.

More blood is taken, more scans, more doctors. No answers.

Three days later, I moved to the renal ward after a discussion between renal and cardiac about who should lead the care for me. Renal led my care, but there were also significant heart concerns, and an echocardiogram showed a build-up of fluid around my heart. I had to go up to the chest ward to have the fluid drained, 400ml to be exact.

No wonder I hadn't been able to walk up those bloody stairs; my heart had been compressed by nearly half a litre of fluid around it.

Suddenly I could feel my heart beating so loudly, I felt a huge relief. This must be the answer, and I must start to get better now.

All sorted?

No such luck: the fluid was a symptom of something else, but what was the cause? This remained "not identified", so off for more blood and scans, and finally a not at all pleasant kidney biopsy.

I promised that this book wouldn't take its self too seriously, and the start of this chapter has been somewhat serious, so I will share two of the lighter conversations during my hospital stay. They say that humour helps in a tricky situation. Well, I tried that; not sure it worked, but they made me laugh at the time. The first was with the chest drain. The lovely Male Irish doctor was getting the large needle ready as the nurses and radiologists were talking to me about the intimacy of what was about to happen and the importance of staying extraordinarily still. The procedure involved an enormous needle going in through the side of my breast while I am still awake and watching, yes indeed not pleasant, not dignified and not funny.

Somehow, we ended up talking about women decorating their private parts with sparkly jewellery. The nurses and I were giggling like teenagers when the consultant came over to do his thing. It was excruciating and not something I could ever recommend. In fact, I have sworn that if ever I need it doing again, I want to be knocked out first with anaesthetic as I cannot go through it awake again.

Calmly, he carries on with the procedure (well he does have a needle a few millimetres from my heart) without a hint that he has listened to the awkward conversation. As he finishes and clears away the bucket of fluid that has been drained from around my heart, he quietly comments that it was not as embarrassing as having lady parts decorated.

I was mortified, I wanted the earth to open and swallow me in one gulp. However, as embarrassing as it was, it really was the perfect distraction from the procedure, and I thank the nurses and radiographer immensely for the conversation and care. And a massive thank you to the consultant for not getting distracted and puncturing my heart with the needle!

The second joke was purely on me, and I am embarrassed that I gave in to such a stereotype, but please understand I was panicking about what was about to happen, and I just started talking! I'm ready for my kidney biopsy, kneeling on all fours in my underwear and a hospital gown, on a table with an x-ray machine pointing through my back. The German consultant is about to stick what I can only describe as an electric meat knife, with a thin blade, in through my back to my kidneys. Here he will remove something the size of "| " or half a cm length of hair. I am told not to move or breathe, as there is a HIGH risk of causing severe bleeding and a small risk of death.

As I am looking at the screen and seeing my innards, I sweetly ask him for some 'High German precision please'. He looked at me as if I was crazy! However, he *was* precise, and I will always be glad for that; even if it is highly embarrassing how I babble on about any strange subject in nerve-wracking situations. I have not learnt anything from this experience: I still talk non-stop when I am nervous and often say inappropriate things to doctors in consultations, and my husband is subsequently embarrassed by me.

Following the biopsy, I had to lie down and not move for six hours. This is not easy, but I was determined not to need a bedpan, so I stuck it out. After five hours, the nurses took pity on me and said I could slowly walk to the bathroom to go to the toilet in private. My stubbornness won out; no peeing in a pot needed.

**Final confirmation**

I was not thrown out of the hospital for racist or crude humour, and finally, after all the poking, prodding, needles in the chest, meat knives in the kidney and other weird tests, I had some answers coming. It was a Friday afternoon; I had been in the hospital for two weeks, and I was desperate to get home to my bed and my bath (and to be home with the family of course, but at that moment the bed and a clean bath came first). I felt slightly better after all the fluid had gone from my heart, but still extremely fragile and exhausted. There were further results to await but no new tests to do, so I could go home and would get a diagnosis within a few days. I felt frustrated that after all that I had gone through, it seemed I was no nearer to the truth. At about 3pm, I walked down to the nurses' station to ask when I was being discharged; I was terrified that if I left it any longer I might miss the Friday afternoon 'window' to escape, and I would have to stay another night if I didn't get the paperwork finished soon. The nurse kindly smiled at me and told me the Doctor was on his way with some medication as they had some results. I asked, 'what results?' but as with so many questions over the last few years, she didn't have the answer, and I had to wait...

After two weeks of tests in the hospital and years of fighting something unknown, I was terrified at the thought of what I was about to be told. Uncontrollably shaking, I returned to my little part of the ward.

**Waiting for results is hard, and remains hard now, it is easy to just put your life on hold, but this doesn't help, you must face the answers as that is the only way to deal with the outcome and move forward.**

I sat on my bed, all packed up and waiting on my own, about to hear what had been making me feel so useless for so long. The German doctor walks over and with "perfect precision" again gets straight down to business telling me the required facts:

> "The initial results from the biopsy are in, further confirmation will follow, but we are 99% certain you have a rare, life-threatening illness."

I needed high dose steroids immediately, and I needed to come back into the clinic on Tuesday for further treatment. The treatment will likely be immune suppression drugs, a type of chemotherapy!

### What????

This was not what I was expecting; I had not seen that news coming. The steroids have many side effects, especially weight gain and mood swings. Oh joy, I am getting horrendous drugs. Apparently, the treatment will last for approximately three to six months. That was my discharge plan. No further information received at this point.

OK, so now I breathe deeply and try to think straight and stay very calm; no silly jokes are coming out of my mouth at this point. This is serious; this is going to be one hell of a battle.

I cry. I cry lots. I cry in front of doctors and in front of my ward mates. I cry on my husband when he comes to take me home. I stop crying so the kids do not see me upset. Again, out comes the smiling face to hide the reality. I cuddle the girls very tightly.

My brain is in overload as I settle into bed that evening. So much to think about: all the side effects, the high chance of the illness returning even once it is under control, the conversation about whether I want more children (as that alters the treatment options); wow, not at all what I expected. No chance of sleep for a few days, even though I am in my own bed and I've had a lovely hot bath to wash all the horrible hospital smell away.

After a couple of days at home, I return to the clinic with my mother-in-law to discuss my treatment. Apparently, because I don't have severe organ damage, I can take the less dangerous drug, called Methotrexate, rather than cyclophosphamide. You can look them up on the NHS Choices website[11]; neither is particularly healthy for you and both have a lengthy list of side effects and increased risks of many other illnesses, notably leukaemia. The conversation goes along the line of, "You just need these and the high dose of steroids for between three to six months, and then you will be in remission, and we will reduce the steroids slowly. However, you will always be at risk of it returning and so will need to visit my clinic for life every six months. Oh, and you will need some more medication to protect your stomach and some more to protect your bones, and oh, your thyroid is not working very well so here are some tablets for that."

All sounded simple. As I waited for 45 minutes at the hospital pharmacy, I cry again, lots, and I did not bother about putting on a brave face in public; just tears.

I had to have blood tests every week at my local hospital and go back to the hospital (a 30-minute journey each way) every fortnight.

**This amount of monitoring is a full-time commitment, it takes over your life, and the energy it takes from you every week is unimaginable. I was exhausted and had a weekly reminder of how ill I was, just approaching the hospital car park made me feel mentally sicker than I did when I wasn't near hospitals, doctors or nurses.** But I reminded myself that it was only going to be for a maximum of six months. My competitive side rose up, and I told everybody I would beat this illness in three months; bring it on!

---

[11] http://www.nhs.uk/pages/home.aspx

I start to feel a strange relief to finally have a name to call this horrible thing that has been bothering me for years; it is nice to have some evidence of a specific illness and be able to prove I am not just making things up or being pathetic. At least something good has come out of all those tests and needles.

I also learnt that I am quite good at crying and even better at hiding it.


**I'm going to fight**

I was so ready to fight this; I had read the stories of how people beat illnesses to come back stronger and made considerable changes in their life. I'd seen the clichéd movies about overcoming adversity and three months wasn't exactly a long time. I would battle and fight and win. Also, I would do it in three months, not three to six months. I can fight, and I will win.

However.

It is quite hard to fight when you are exhausted and don't fully understand the thing you are battling. As I have said it is rare (in Europe this is defined as 1 in 2000 people according to the Rare Illness network), my GP had never had a patient with it ever (I'm not one to guess ages, but he is definitely over 50 ☺).

There is a brilliant patient association with great material, but it is a complicated illness to understand. I stayed positive, well at least 80% of the time. I talked to people about all of it, and I took some time (two more weeks) off work to rest. My GP signed me back to work, but only if I worked from home as the drugs reduced (suppressed) my immune system, so I was at risk of catching anything flying about. I worked, I rested, and I cuddled my family.

Three months came and went. Four months came and went, and I did feel better than I had before treatment, but I did not feel great. Six months came and went; my blood tests showed all was ok, and chest x-rays were clear, but I still was not right. It felt like a cruel déjà vu, but with many medical tests between the repeated memories. The consultant told me I was not ill and that we all have "minor issues", and that I just had to live with them! He talked about links between mental attitude and physical health. I thought he was implying the symptoms were partly in my head; I took offence at this and felt hurt at the insinuation. I felt so bothered by his comments, in short, I did misunderstand him in this conversation, but he did not try to correct the misunderstanding.

I felt heartbroken. I had been so relieved when the doctors had found an 'identifiable illness' that could explain my weird symptoms, that I was not making it up and that what I felt was real. Yet here I was six months down the line being told the same thing: you just have to live with it. More tears but in private this time; I would not cry in front of this consultant ever again. I could never expose my true feelings after his comments, another person to show that I am fighting and staying 100% positive. Another person I will always have to put a brave face on for.

**I'm not winning**

The realisation that I wasn't getting back to being me took a while to sink in. I sat down in front of my GP explaining again how 'I just don't feel right' because, as the consultant had told me, the mental and physical are closely linked and that maybe the mind was preventing the physical from recovery. If I am honest, I took this to mean that the consultant thought I did not want to get better; this hurt me deeply. I was a fighter, and I was determined to win; how dare he question my attitude. Looking back, I don't think I helped the situation because I held it together and stayed strong most of the time. As soon as I went into the consulting room at the hospital, the relief at being able to talk about it to somebody who I thought would fully understand how I felt, meant I cried a fair bit in that room with him. It was the only place I felt I could be honest about how I felt during the long struggle, it was a safe place for me to not try and be brave, a place to really explain everything I was facing.

I really was not winning this battle. Most mornings after I had dropped the children at school, I would curl into bed with my laptop and work while trying desperately to keep my head upright. When my husband was away at work, I would curl back into my bed as soon as the children were in their beds at 7pm. Mine was a well-used bed (and not in a fun way). I took the blame for this failure to recover on myself. I know that is not logical, but I could not get the comment about mental and physical links out of my head. I thought that somehow, I must be blocking my recovery from the physical and genuine illness, by not fighting hard enough or not resting enough or something else that I had no idea about. I felt I was losing my fight, and I had lost the person I could really explain this too, so I struggled on.

I went back and asked for anti-depressants again, as I really did not know what else to do anymore. The fight within me was dying; I just didn't have the energy.

I didn't stay on the anti-depressants long as I realised that this was a load of bullshit and there was nothing wrong in my brain, other than being confused, frustrated, a little too ambitious and impatient. **I had lost confidence in my ability to judge what was going on, but I still knew I was not making all this up. There was still something wrong with me physically; I just knew it.**

I had a very long conversation with my Doctor friend, and again, she steered me in the right direction. I researched the best hospitals for my illness and found that one of the leading places in the world was just an hour away. I was not winning at this moment, and I had totally lost confidence in my consultants, so I requested my GP transfer me to another hospital. I think it is safe to say that, for me, it probably saved my life. I felt very positive about being proactive and trying to find solutions. Mentally I felt more in control; physically, I was still in pieces and suffering terribly. But I had stepped away from feeling that it was me preventing the healing and that I was doing something wrong, I had a severe illness, and it would take time to heal and that I would recover in my own time and in my own way. **It would not work to a perfect schedule outlined by somebody else. I had to face my issues my way and find the right people to support me, just because somebody has a title; it does not guarantee that they will always be** right. **If you doubt a decision made about your health, challenge it or ask for a second or even third opinion.**

I think at this stage I only felt marginally better physically than I had before treatment, and yet I had taken high dose toxic medicines for nearly a year; it was soul destroying and impossible to keep trying to live normally.

Once I had found the correct 'Centre of Excellence', I went and talked to my GP and asked for a referral; he reluctantly completed the paperwork. You have a right to request this in the UK. **Make sure you know your rights; you have a right to choose where to be seen**. **Do a little research online to find the right experts.** Full details of your rights can be found here: **https://www.gov.uk/government/publications/the-nhs-choice-framework**


**I cannot cope any longer with this fight**

I waited for my new appointment to come through with the 'Centre of Excellence'. I found it increasingly hard to deal with so many aspects of still feeling ill. Some outward issues, like what do you say when people utter the line, 'how are you?' or when they tell you that 'you look so well … considering', or 'I should just be glad it's not cancer', or 'don't worry about the added weight, we all know it is down to the drugs, and it isn't really you'…. So many things that people say while they are trying to be kind, which make you feel so very sad. These were from friends who I loved and cared deeply for.

I know they were trying to make me feel better, but I just withdrew, as I didn't know how to deal with the questions or comments. And all made me want to do was cry again. I don't know what I wanted them to say, maybe just a cuddle, all I know is that I didn't have an answer to their questions. I really didn't know what to say, I knew if I said more than a simple sentence I would burst into tears, and I know that wasn't the response my friends were looking for when they asked the questions.

Daily I found it hard to get out of bed, to face life, to smile, to shower or just to care about me. I still do this now when I am having a tough time. I withdraw and just hide away; it is easier, but it does not really help. A couple of my old friends can spot this, even though they are not physically close. They detect the lack of posts on Facebook or the late birthday presents; it is good to have friends who 'just kind of know'.

Don't get me wrong, my children are washed, fed, cleaned and loved, but after caring for the girls, I have nothing left. I had totally lost my fight and self-concern. More coffee was needed each morning. I was exhausted and did not know how to cope with anything anymore. I did keep working because from behind a laptop, nobody can see your emotions, so I used words like 'love, passion, enthusiasm' in my emails and totally masked my real emotional state. I smiled nicely on the 15 minutes of the school run, and people told me they admired my fight and strength and that I was an inspiration. I was hiding this all brilliantly, again the master of hiding behind my smile.

Writing this makes it sound like I hid all my feelings on purpose and that it was all a sinister master plan. As with many things in our lives, that isn't true. I hadn't planned my response to any of this; I just found my own personal way of coping. It was not really a healthy way of dealing with issues, as I became increasingly withdrawn. Friends pulled gently away; always a bit too busy to have that coffee with me, not enough money to go out. When my husband travelled with work, I gave up inviting people over; I just sat watching mindless TV and then going to bed early.

The working from home that had been a blessing at the beginning by allowing me to carry on working now made it easy for me to hide and not really have a proper conversation with people for days at a time.

My husband had taken on a big job (to ensure our security), so he was doing very long hours with many nights away. I got lost somewhere between the normal world and a new sad world where I felt so dreadful every day that I wanted to hide in bed. **It was like I was standing in no-mans land, with my healthy self on one side and sick me** from the hospital on the other, but I was no longer either of those people, I had changed and didn't feel like I belonged on either side.

**I was lonely and felt like I was drowning**.

We had lost our fabulous dog to cancer, and I really missed him. I missed him by my side, I missed the need to go out for daily walks, and I just felt lonely without him. It is tough to write this, and I have tears brewing; the loneliness was unbearable, even though I had my children and husband who loved me, and I loved them, and I saw people every day.

**But I couldn't share everything with them**.

After years of being ill, you cannot keep going on about it to friends and family. Everybody has their own issues, and there is a time when your chronic illness just gets boring for others. I was aware of this and hated discussing the problems I faced, but I was screaming inside, desperate to talk to somebody. That big screaming voice drove me to write this book. I tried to find things to read to help me understand and cope, but I didn't see anything that explained the lengthy battle that dealing with a condition for life brings. I saw many books on specific illnesses, but, for me, my struggle is less with the physical symptoms and more with the consequences of the physical symptoms.

**I found the loneliness and helplessness very hard; I so wanted life to go back to being normal but did not have the first clue of how to do that**.

**Life must change**

When we are hit with momentous change, we need to go on living, and we need to find a way of accepting our current life. This isn't easy, and it will take each of us a different amount of time, or a different number of triggers, to start the change. My change was the realisation of a simple sentence:

**No work, friend or colleague will remember that I let him or her down in ten years, but my family will never forget if I am not around.**

This probably sounds a little melodramatic, and maybe it is, but I had been trying to do everything and be there for everybody. My change came from realising that I need to look after myself in order to look after my family. If I push myself to go to meetings and end up exhausted in bed for a month, that doesn't help anybody. On the other hand, if I give in and withdraw that leaves me low and miserable, which again does not help anybody.

My life changed: I started to put myself first. I don't mean that I ran off to a retreat for months on end; I mean I made small readjustments to make sure I looked after myself so that, in turn, I could look after my family. I started Yoga, I cut down on alcohol, and I tried to eat a little more healthily. Just some small changes; no drastic plans like never eating carbs again or only eating fruit on weekdays. Within a few months, my symptoms had not gone, but I did feel brighter, and people made genuine comments that I looked good, note: none of the extra comments at the end of the compliments, i.e. you look good **considering** what you are going through. Whoop whoop! It felt good. I started making time to read books that interested me and spent time learning things I wished I had studied harder at school.

My illness is still there, and always will be. I will always be wondering if I am having a flare or is it just a simple cold, but I cannot let it ruin mine and my family's life; I must find a way to keep some normality throughout all this craziness.

There are many books and 'experts' who can tell you how to be happy. They never really rang true for me, and now I understand why. We are all different and what makes us happy is very different, so this book won't give you a tick list of how to 'get back to living normally'. However, I believe you should take some time to realise what you enjoy or what makes your brain spark. You know that feeling when you see something, and you MUST read it, or you MUST have a go at something. It could be anything. For my eldest, it is anything to do with dogs or horses; for my youngest, it is dancing and dragons from 'how to train your dragon'. It is about finding things that don't feel like hard work or that you could do for hours without realising the time has passed, for me, it was dog walking, reading and drawing.

To deal with my chronic illness, I needed to find something that I loved doing.

I know we have an everyday life to deal with: finances, mortgages, family, ironing, work and housework…. Sometimes it feels overwhelming to do it all, and this is where the priorities need to shift. **Get help if you can. Do not think that doing something you like is selfish or wasting your short supply of energy**; you need these enjoyable experiences to keep positive, and when we are positive, everything else seems a little easier.

One shift I made was to switch from watching TV, which was not interesting, to spending more time reading books that interested me. The same amount of effort was needed, but the reading made me feel happy, whereas watching most TV programmes left me feeling empty.

I bought a step tracker and tried to walk over 7000 steps a day (I know the recommendation is 10,000, but I found if I did this every day, I was exhausted) to give me that little extra motivation to get my butt moving.

One thing you should NOT do: read health, fitness or beauty magazines; they are depressing if you are fit and healthy, full of unattainable perfection. If you start reading these when feeling unwell, it is even harder to stomach … throw them all in the bin. Most of us are not models, so why are we comparing ourselves to these people? In the current world of male grooming and fashion, I think this point now applies to both male and females. My daughters and I love the Anita Roddick, The Body Shop founder, quote that there are 8 million women in the world and only 8 who look like supermodels.

My big switch was my attitude to work: I dropped it down in my priorities. I still worked hard and did my job well, but not at the cost of my family or my health. This meant I had a little more energy at home and a little more time to cuddle my family or read with the girls. I also managed to persuade my husband to get a puppy (this took some real persuasion), so I now had company again through the day and a reason to go out and keep my legs moving.

I know when you read this, you will think, "well, that is ok for her but…." Only you know what 'buts' you will add in there, and that's fine, you need to find your way of coping. I know it is hard and only when you are ready will you push those 'buts' aside and make some changes that help you.

It took me years to feel like I could start living again and I still have some days where I don't want to be full of life; then I withdraw for a day or two (sometimes longer). That's my solitude time, my time to think and re-gather my priorities. Please just realise there are small things you can do to get your passion back. They do not need to take lots of time or energy, but they should be something you LOVE.

One last comment on fighting back: **don't force it.** When we have a life-shaking event, we need time to process it and come to terms mentally and physically before we can start to get back to living. For some people, this may be a few weeks or months, or for others, like me, it can take years. There is no correct way to process all this, no handbook or timetable of when you should do things. Remember that some days you'll feel that you have made progress and yet the next day you may feel you haven't progressed at all. I think this is normal; well, that's what I tell myself, as I regularly have days when I think I'm not moving forward!

Change at your own pace, but please do try to make some positive changes. The alternative is not a happy place to be.

### Life can still be good

When I wrote this section heading, I was in a happy place. However, it has been a section that I have looked at and thought I'm not ready to write that yet.

Why?

I think the reason it is difficult to write and think about is that it's not the 'good' I had always thought of as good. 'Good' is subjective and can mean many things; this makes it hard to define simply, but also gives us a wonderful opportunity to make 'good' whatever we want it to be for ourselves. Chronic illness can force us to step back from our lives, this stepping back from normal life can put us in a privileged position that not everybody gets to see. It allows us to watch the world around us, and think, and see what is valuable in our lives.

When I have bad days, it is a strange feeling as it allows me to sit back and watch the world and those in it and observe it from a different angle, watching the world rush past. It is a unique perspective, and over the years, I have used this to my advantage to really take time out and evaluate what is critical and what are my priorities. It is almost like a time to look at how to shape your future, and the good that you can see in these moments may not be what you always thought good was. For me, in these timeout moments, I go for walks, garden and read, and do these things at a leisurely pace instead of trying to fit them in between everything else. A time to walk away from the stress of life and slow down, I may feel dreadful in these moments, but my brain enjoys the change of pace for a short time.

When you have a restriction on something, it pushes you to plan how to manage the resources you do have. For example, if you are a bit lacking in finances, you sit back and take stock: what do you have, what is coming in, what you must spend money on and what is nice to spend money on with the resources you have. Then you try to make it all balance; this isn't always easy, and it forces you to prioritise those items you <u>must have</u> over those that are <u>nice to have</u>.

It is the same when you have compromised health. You are not balancing the financial books this time, you are adjusting your health and energy levels; if you cannot do it all, then you **must** choose your priorities.

I am 40+ and, if I am honest, before this last few years, I thought I would live forever and never have to think about losing my energy or things going wrong; well not at least till I was 80. Naïve, I know. Now I find that every day I must prioritise what I spend my energy on, which sounds depressing and it can get you down. But if you are smart about the planning, it can open a new world where you prioritise the things that you genuinely love. Having compromised energy levels has a way of sharpening your brain, you don't want to waste your energy on things which do not bring you pleasure. I like to focus on things that I love and have a passion for, we have so many things we try to get done that we rarely think about what we really love to do when we have a choice.

This is where life can get better.

**Write down the things you must do, like cleaning, ironing and cooking, and then work out which of these make you happy and which leave you either exhausted or dreading them. Next, find a solution for the ones you dread or the tasks that make you feel exhausted**; for me, it was ironing my husband's work shirts and cleaning. My answer was to send the work shirts to the dry cleaners, it was about £10 a week, but it saved me a couple of hours. Also, we got a cleaner that came once a week for two hours. These sound like luxury things, and they are, but there is a real benefit: if you can take away the things that really leave you tired, you can fit in the fun stuff or continue to work the selected hours if you enjoy your work (which is what I did).

If money is an issue, talk to your partner, children, or friends and see if they can help. I found that my eldest was desperate to assist in the kitchen and hoover (for free), but I had been too busy to realise this. Now she helps me, setting the table, tidying afterwards or washing up… as a famous supermarket says 'every little helps'. My youngest is now the Cutlery Queen: she sets out the cutlery for meals and empties the cutlery from the dishwasher. She is very proud of her title and, although it does not sound like much, some days it really is a relief when she helps me with these small tasks.

It could be a matter of re-assessing. Fewer cappuccinos a month could mean a cleaner coming in once a month just for a thorough one-off clean, which leaves you with more energy to re-pot that plant you have wanted to do for the last two months.

I found a nice quote which rings true for me:

*We must be willing to let go of the life we have planned,*

*so as to accept the life that is waiting for us.*

*Joseph Campbell, American Author*

This is hard, and if you find out how to completely let go of the old life, please let me know (as I'm still clinging on to some parts of my past life). It is useful to think that we have to say goodbye to some things to let us have space for the new things that come into our life. This is natural and happens to everybody throughout our life. For example, how many of the fun things we did at primary school do we still do in our sensible grown-up life? Not many. However, this is a gradual, natural change over many years, so we accept the change. When we suddenly find we have an illness and are FORCED to change, we push back on this forced change and see it as entirely negative. We need to try and find positives in our forced changes and use the switch to make some welcome adjustments to the life we are living.

I am not saying that having a chronic illness is brilliant for you. Not at all, but I do think that life continues and that to have a happy life, the best thing we can do is readjust and find a way to live with the changes. My life is better now in so many ways, but yes, I miss going for a run, or partying all night, or even just being active without the knowledge that I will really suffer over the next few days. Instead, I enjoy the relaxed time with my children, I ditched the things I detest, I found out which of my friends are real friends, and I re-found my love of reading.

**In general, I stopped pretending to be somebody else and started being me, and it was a version of me that I had not really thought about when I had been running around trying to be 'successful'.**

The primary reason life is good now is that I made the decision to appreciate and prioritise family, my fantastic husband and my gorgeous girls. I look at the girls and sometimes wonder if I will be there when they get married or will I be a Grandma. Who knows, but I now make decisions based on what gives me the best chance of seeing them both become the amazing adults I know they will become. So yes, life is good; different, but good.

**Knockbacks will always happen.**

Everybody has knockbacks; these are part of everyday life. The problem is that when you have a chronic illness and you have a down day, you very quickly blame the illness, it is an easy scapegoat. The fact that you have this debilitating illness seems to make any negative occurrences, either physical or mental, harder to deal with, and it can make us over-react. Maybe it is because we are tired or the influence of drugs we take, or maybe it is simply that our health becomes such a big part of our daily life. When I find myself blaming the illness, my husband calmly comments that these things happened before, and I took them in my stride and managed to cope ;-).

When my cholesterol went (a little) above the recommended levels, I panicked that the illness caused it, and I was going to get steroid-induced diabetes... arrrrrgggghhhhhh. Days of worrying and more crying.

STOP.

In the cold light of day when I had eventually calmed down, I thought about why. It was probably down to the fact that I had been forced to stop exercising, and for months during treatment, I hadn't left the house. Both of which had meant I had put on a couple of stone (with a little additional help from the infamous steroids) and had not been moving very much, except between the fridge, the sofa and my lovely warm bed. Of course, this would influence the cholesterol. So once calm, I gradually increased the walking and cut back on takeaways and crisps. Lo and behold, within a couple of months, I had lost some weight, and the cholesterol had reduced to below the level of concern. No big miracle, just thinking about what I would have done if faced with the issue before I had the illness.

The knockbacks don't have to be related to the illness, but they could be. I know that each time I have any medical tests I dread receiving the results, and if they prove to be not what you want to hear, it's hard to deal with it; it is hard to wait for results. It is challenging to continue with normal life when you feel like you are continually awaiting results, but you must. Take the knockback; whatever it is, cry, wallow, shout, whatever it is that allows you to process it in your brain, then look with cold, hard, factual eyes and decide what to do or how to adjust to the changes. Talk to your GP, and if they are not good support, find a helpful doctor. It is your right to request a change of GP to one who will support you and your family. Talk to friends or family, just please do not hide away for too long. Face it, and you will be able to deal with it. Facing it will not make it go away, but it can help you to decide how to cope with it.

**You need to take the emotion out of results, talk to somebody, GP, family or friend who can look at the results as simple facts and try to review in an unemotional manner.**

With regards to work, explaining results can be difficult, going back and informing your boss can add stress to the relationship. I have found an effective way of dealing with my boss: every time I go and see a doctor, I sleep on the conversation before I discuss it with him. I need overnight space to process the news, whether it is good or bad. Sleep puts things into perspective for me. He thinks this is very funny, but it works for us and allows me to discuss things calmly. When I first became ill, I would call and update him as soon as I came out of appointments, frequently with tears in my eyes. I would try to explain all the details when I didn't really know what I was trying to say because I had not sorted all the information out or deciphered what it meant to me. I use the same sleep-on-it rule for replying to work emails that annoy me or that I don't know how to deal with. I leave them overnight, and my subconscious works out a solution – I really recommend this as a tool for coping with knockbacks.

The process of leaving things overnight allows me to remove some of the emotion and focus on the facts saving my boss from having to listen to me ramble on for 30 minutes with no real point to what I am saying. Once I have processed the events, I can typically summarise it in a few minutes. The same with social media: really have a think before you post any updates about your struggles. Make sure you are doing it for the right reasons and remember all your 'friends' and 'friends of friends and future employers' can read the comments. If you want to be selective about who will read your details, send a direct message to a group of friends rather than a public posting.

I suffered a significant knockback when, after a year of the 'new wonder drug', my illness returned stronger. This was hard for me to deal with, and it felt like somebody had taken away all my future; I had such a strong emotional reaction. More tears, a few days hiding away and a few more books read, and then coffee with a kind friend helped me to process all the emotions. If I am honest, I did not want to go for coffee, as I felt so incredibly tired and weak and emotionally fragile, but I knew (somewhere deep down) that it would help, and I should now allow friends in and talk to them. I had a large cappuccino, a gorgeous gooey muffin and I giggled (and cried a little) and giggled, and I left the coffee shop with a big hug and a smile on my face. This was the first smile in days. Coffee and cake will not solve the physical problems, but emotionally, I felt so much stronger: ready to start my battle again.

**So why not every time you have any kind of knockback, wallow a little, let it process, review the facts, then get out and face the world with a smile and maybe a big gooey muffin.**

### Planning

I now plan more, and I plan less than before I gained an illness.

Day to day I plan more: I anticipate how much I think I can do in a day and work out my priorities; I think about what I have coming up in the next few days, will it be the weekend? Do I need to conserve energy for the kids? Do I have a friend's birthday coming up? All this now requires more planning to make sure I can be present at the major events in my life.

However, I now plan a lot less for the future; not in a depressing, 'I'm going to die' way. I mean I think about where we would like to go on holiday, but I do not book things too far in advance anymore, 'just in case'. I do not book too many physical business meetings, as I do not know if I will make it on the day. After having to cancel so many nights out, meetings or weekends at friends, I now prefer to arrange things closer to the time rather than let people down by cancelling. I am not sure all my friends really understand this, and some may think I am distant, but it is my way of coping.

For me, one of the hardest things about living with an illness which causes fatigue is cancelling on people. It goes against every bone in my body; I feel like I am failing and letting people down. Most people in my life do understand now, but I still really struggle with this aspect of the illness.

So now I plan more for the short-term and less for the long-term, with one exception: I plan financially and legally in detail for the long-term; I may not be here in the future, but I need to know that my family is protected should something happen. Luckily, I had taken out a life insurance plan before I became ill; it costs me £10 a month but will pay off the mortgage should the worst happen. Also, my work benefits and pension will help significantly, but I am aware that there may be a time when I cannot continue to work.

Recently we met with a financial adviser to ensure coverage for that and any other future events.

One more thing you really should do if you have not already, draw up a legal Will. I am not implying we are all going to drop dead tomorrow, but I have found it a great relief to know I have sorted things out for my family both legally and financially. Also, it allows a great joke with my husband that I am worth more dead than alive ... although I think I find this funnier than he does.

Another area you need to plan carefully is the supply of medication. Never leave any of this until the last minute, I have run out of steroids before, and it really is not fun. I order my repeat prescriptions online through the surgery website and keep them all in a big box, and then once or twice a month I measure them all out into individual small am and pm boxes. This allows me to track which medications are running low, but it also means I only must think about the number of drugs I take once or twice a month.

Most days, I just throw them down my throat in one go; this really helps my mental state as it only takes 30 seconds a day.

Remember you need extra for Christmas, Easter and holidays. I know this is obvious when you read it, but I bet we have all forgotten the additional prescriptions at Christmas. For holidays, I take my repeat prescription forms and my medication in my hand luggage and have never had a problem with customs this way, even when travelling to Washington, D.C., USA.

This chapter and its subsections have run through the phases I faced; it is just how things happened to me and what I learnt along the way. I want to share my story because I wish somebody had told me all the stuff that came with a chronic illness up front when I was first diagnosed. Not just the impacts of the disease on the body but how its tentacles spread into every part of who you are and how you live. I am no expert, and you will face different and maybe more or less challenging issues, but hopefully, you can see that there are ways to cope.

This is not an easy journey, and I am not perfect at driving down the roads.

**I don't manage to follow my own advice all the time, but I figure if I can stick to the 80:20 rule, following the rules 80% of the time, I will be doing well. The main lesson is not to be too hard on ourselves when we lose control.**

# Talking about 'it.'

I have two beautiful young children at school. I love them very much, but one thing I have not enjoyed doing during all the stages of my illness is school drop off and pick up. What do you say to people EVERY DAY???? That's every day, people asking you the same questions, every day. Initially, I retreated; I was probably quite rude, but I couldn't cope with going over everything several times a day when I didn't really understand any of what was happening myself. How could I explain it to others in a five-minute conversation at the school gate? Do people really want to know that your insides feel like they have been ripped out and put in a blender and shoved back inside? And should I really be describing this in front of your, mine or any other peoples' children?

I couldn't, and I didn't want to; I'm not prepared to share my suffering every day. I also found that if I kept repeating how awful I felt, I would find myself getting really upset, and that isn't too healthy for anybody. And it certainly does not win friends. It was almost as if the more I talked about the facts, the worse I felt, like some strange self-fulfilling prophecy. However, on the flip side, I don't want to tell everybody that I feel great because I didn't, I felt dreadful, and I need these friends to understand this; not just for my sake, but also for my children's. The children are undeniably affected by the illness, nearly as much as I am; they need support and help as this is too much for them to face alone. So, what to do? How to meet my friends every day and not pretend all is great or that I am going to drop dead at any moment, as in reality, they are just trying to be helpful? What to do?

**Have a strategy. Plan in advance.**

Not a big three-year business-plan or a complicated mission statement; something simple, something you would naturally say, something that means I'm doing ok, but the illness is still all going on inside. Maybe you cannot see it, but it is still there shouting very loudly at me. I chose a concise and straightforward statement (a little like me, my husband started our wedding speech with the statement 'I will keep this short and simple like my new wife' – how charming?) that would not make anybody feel awkward but didn't ignore their questions:

> I'm fine today thanks, how are you?

So simple, so short and from my perspective, what it was really saying was:

> I'm not great but don't really want to talk about things here, and now, please tell me something happy from your side to make me smile.

It worked, most of the time. It allowed people to move on to happier conversations, but with the feeling that they did the friend thing and asked me how I was. Some friends will push you for more; I'm not sure about how this makes me feel. It is hard to say that you don't feel any better than last week and you don't really expect to see any improvement over the next few years unless some wonderful miracle cure (that you cannot let yourself dream about) is found that takes it all away. Nobody wants to hear that at 8.50am. Yet, some friends will hope and expect to see you continually improving. I think this is human nature; they want the best for you and cannot understand why this is not happening. Friends expect to see you on an upwards curve improving all the time when it is a very unpredictable wiggly line, often flat with no upward trend. When you are ready, you could sit down with these friends and explain it clearly and help them to understand that you may never fully recover and may be left with many reminders of the treatment and the journey you are going through with the illness.

I hope that any of my friends reading this will not take my strategy as a negative way to deal with their concerned questions; it was never meant to be that. The approach is there to prevent me from bursting into tears or stop me from constantly repeating the most depressing words I have ever heard again and again and again. I do believe in the concept that if you talk about the worst things that can happen, then they will eventually happen.

My strategy got me through a lot of days waiting on the school playground, trying to hold it all together without crying. I know my actions were strange for friends because it left some of them not really knowing whether to ask how you feel, and that is fine. One friend said a lovely thing after she had asked me how I was. She merely giggled and said, "what a stupid question. From now on, I am just going to say hello and not keep asking you." It made me realise that it is complicated for friends to say the right thing. We need to understand that it is hard for friends to see us every day and do the usual flippant 'you ok?' It is such a natural comment that comes out automatically. Therefore, I realise that some comments may hurt us or make us feel useless, but 99% of the time no hurt is intended. It is just a lack of understanding, or an automatic comment said to anybody; try not to take the comments personally.

On days when more information gushed out of my mouth – and it did – I generally cried through the words, because once the emotional control is interrupted, it all came out. Everything. When I used my set statement, I held it together and often did get a laugh because of my friend's silly stories. A simple, clear strategy and little forward planning can lead to the difference between crying in front of the children and them seeing you laughing, but with your friends knowing all was NOT great. Perfect.

The above is excellent for the public interaction with friends, but in private with close friends, the last thing you should do is pretend or hold it all in. Human nature is about communities and friendships, and when something significant happens, you need to lean on friends. You need to share the problems and the humorous parts of the illness (and there will be some), as well as your fears; just talk, talk and talk. I found it easy to speak at the beginning, to explain everything and sort of enjoy receiving the sympathy hugs and kisses; having a rare illness somehow felt special, it felt interesting. People were desperate to hear all about it: I shared my fun 'one-liner', how my GP has never had a patient with this in his 20 years, how the consultant who couldn't work out what was happening was called Dr Mystry. All fun, entertaining stories. However, after six years the stories are old and boring and, as I don't really get out and about much, I don't really have many funny stories, other than flippant comments from the kids, or my numerous trips to hospitals.

After a period, you start to wonder how many more times you can bore friends; some back away quite quickly, and I suggest you just let these people drift away. Don't get upset by these people. There may be many reasons for their drifting away, maybe they have issues of their own and cannot fit anybody else's problems in, or perhaps they are terrified of illness and are scared to talk to you. Whatever the reason, don't take it personally and just let them go. Trying to keep up the friendship will only lead to hurt for you; it is easier to accept that the link is gone.

Real friends will still be there after three years, five years or however long it is, and will always try and understand all the twists and turns. But please remember, and this is a tough one, the world does not revolve around our illness; other things are happening, and other people have problems. It is easy to fall into the belief that you have it far worse than anybody else. We still need to be a friend to friends, and that doesn't mean that we just always talk about the illness. This isn't easy, especially if the illness is not under control, and you are really struggling. It is easy to fall into being a selfish friend who forgets to ask about others. Friends have two-way conversations; both get support and a chance to moan.

A conversation about something completely different could possibly make you giggle and laugh and transport you to a world where there is no illness. Try it. Try having a good gossip and laugh about something a bit naughty or racy over a glass of something; forget the world. It will help. I think part of the trick is to not wait around for a cure or the next test results but to live for now. I believe that if a patient is told they have a temporary issue, they can sit and wait for it to be gone, but if they are told it is permanent, they are more likely to get on with life and deal with the issues. One of my favourite quotes (and it hangs in my downstairs toilet) is:

> *Do not dwell in the past, do not dream of the future, concentrate the mind on the present moment.*
>
> **Buddha**

## What can you do now to make your life easier?

When my fatigue hits, I find it very easy to hide away and tell everybody I am too tired to talk; I retreat. On the occasions that I force myself to go out and see people, it really helps, and I find that I bounce back quicker. Having young children helps with this as I must leave the house each morning to get them to school, but if you don't have that as a reason, you must find a way to get out and about. Moving, walking, and fresh air will lift you, even if you walk at a snail's pace, and can only manage 15 minutes. This is enough to give you a boost of vitamin D, get the muscles working and give you a little cardio workout. I can recommend a dog to get you moving, as each day you must take them out, and each night they will snuggle up with you and keep you warm. One of my biggest knocks came when my gorgeous Labrador had to be put to sleep. In one go, I lost my exercise partner, my sounding board, my relaxation toy… my amazing friend. I tried hard to persuade my husband to get a puppy, but he thought the extra work would be too much and, as he is ever sensible, maybe he had a point. But I so wanted my baby back.

## Talking to children about your illness

Talking with my children is one of the hardest parts of my having a chronic illness. Children understand things at face value. If they get sick mummy gives them a magic kiss, a coloured plaster or the genius of Calpol, all of which work perfectly, and they get better. The 'get better' is the part that they understand, so if you don't get fully better it is hard for them to work out why and to process the implications of this 'not getting better'. Does it mean that the doctors and the drugs have failed? Does it mean you will get worse and eventually die? If you stay poorly, tired and unable to play like you used to, it is easy for them to feel like they are the ones suffering through all this. My eldest used to say, "when can we go running around the playground together again?" This hurt; no matter how 'sensibly' I look at this statement, it still hurts.

I want my children to stay children as long as possible. At this moment, I can shield them from a lot of my symptoms, and I use my precious energy reserves to ensure they have as normal a life as possible. This has been, and always will be, my priority. They know I am ill and that I sleep more than their friends' parents do; they understand that they cannot jump on me as I am too fragile, that I cannot chase them around the garden or lift them up, but, this doesn't really upset them. I still cuddle and kiss them and read with them and make them do their homework and guitar practice.

Talking to your children is a very personal conversation and one that should not be blown up into a big issue; the more significant the fuss you make, the scarier it will seem to both you and your children. I believe the most critical aspect is to be honest. This does not, however, mean that you need to go into every little tiny detail about the illness, the risks associated with the illness and the subsequent treatment. Remember you are talking to a child who has minimal worldly experience and takes the words at 'face value', often without being able to read the full message behind the words. I have found that it helps me if I have a few days to process whatever news it is I am going to tell my children before I tell them. This means the emotion has left me, and I am ready to discuss just the facts without the extra irrelevant sensational parts.

It is a very different conversation from the one with your partner or friends when you want to tell them everything and gain some sympathy/support out of them; a discussion with your Child is about keeping things clear and simple, not getting too emotional and listening to their concerns.

I found it easier to discuss possible symptoms that I may face up front with my children as I thought this would help prevent them being surprised, one of which was the potential to lose my hair when I started chemotherapy. My daughters were four and nine, so one wanted to be a princess, and the other wanted to start shopping in trendy shops and buy accessories; not the perfect time to mention that mum might become bald. However, having discussed it with the GP I believed (and still do) that it would be better to chat about it before it happened, than for my daughters to come into the bedroom one morning and find lots of hair on my pillow. So, one day, while I was finishing the first French plait of the morning, I gently discussed the side effects of the upcoming treatment: tiredness, weakness and the possibility that I could lose my hair. I just quietly slipped it in there. After a moment's pause, I suggested that I would need some serious help in choosing scarves to make sure that my bald head would stay warm, as daddy would be dreadful at picking smart ones. They giggled and decided orange would be good, and the conversation was completed.

Over the next few days, I had a few questions from the nine-year-old; mostly about which shops we would go to, but also about whether it was happening yet. It never happened. However, I do not regret bringing it up. I'd removed significant stress for me, and it taught my children a lot about appearance and how, if you see a bald person maybe, just maybe, something is going on that you don't know about. My children made me very proud (again) with the way they handled all the information and uncertainty.

Working closely with the school really does help to keep the information factual and ensure that the girls face the same message both at home and school. On the odd occasion, it got too much for my eldest, the school considered the circumstances surrounding any 'outbursts' that were out of character. The school and I both explained that any such behaviour is not acceptable, and the punishment for breaking the school rules stood, but a little extra support for talking about feelings was put into place. I live in an area where children take the 11+, and at nine, my daughter was right at the start of thinking about these exams and her choice of secondary school. I was conscious that my illness should not impact on the decisions we made together. The focus was very much on ensuring that her effort was on work and was not interrupted. I didn't want my daughters to use my illness as an excuse to get bad grades and mess around, we were to carry on as close to normal as possible.

The downside of being honest about what is happening is that they will worry (maybe not the very young one, who thinks a blanket, a cuddle and watching Disney's Frozen solves everything – and it does go a long way to solving the world's problems). As a parent or grandparent, you need to be there to hear the worries and respond. I have tried not to say, 'oh don't worry, it will all be perfect'; I promised them I wouldn't lie. I have explained that I will never return to full health, that I will always have some damage and the possibility of a major flare of the illness, but I am hopeful of returning to a more normal way of life. This is what I explain, that we do many fun things as a family, but that yes, we do have some limitations. It is a difficult conversation, but it seems to stop my daughters' imaginations running away and visualising an unpleasant future.

One teacher hadn't really understood all the implications of the illness, and after I had finished a course of treatment, she warmly told my daughter, 'look mummy is all better now'. I didn't make any comments at that moment but spoke with her later, explaining that I would prefer not to imply that all was great and cured now; she accepted this going forward. Separately I chatted with the girls and this time I pinched an idea from a wonderful nurse I meet at the clinic. **I explained that the illness is like a volcano: it was currently dormant, but it is still there and could erupt in the future, or it may stay dormant for a while. If it came back, it might be a large-scale eruption or a little hiccup of fire.** This helped the children understand that it will always be there, but it shouldn't rule our lives because it could stay controlled and therefore, we can live with it. This conversation helped them to visualise the volcano, and it made them giggle to think of Mummy erupting like a volcano.

How will I tell them if the end approaches? I'm not sure, but I hope I continue along the same path and that I can be honest, factual and supportive to them, as they are the main priority in my life, and I love them very much. I think they will grow stronger whatever happens over the next few years and I hope they live all their dreams to the maximum. At every opportunity, that is the message they get from me!

You know your children and grandchildren better than anybody else; just be honest with them in the way you think they can cope with and be there to listen when they get scared or intrigued. Remember that words are not the only way that we talk to people, our body language and actions play a significant part. A hug will always help more than a thousand words, and I do love a good squeeze.

Good luck with your own conversations, it is not an easy one.

# Pacman

I read about the spoon theory[12]. I thought it was terrific and understood how it could help many people like me. In short, you have a set number of spoons per day and each activity uses them up, for example, getting dressed could use up one spoon. So, by the end of the day, if you have been out and about, you don't have any spoons left to go dancing or even chatting with your partner.

Over the last few years, while this has helped me, it didn't seem to ultimately add up, as some days I feel I have more spoons to use and some days I feel like I only have a teaspoon left by the time I reach lunchtime. I thought there must be something that influences the energy; I am not suggesting some ridiculous strict fruit juicing or no-carbs diet, I don't believe in either, but I do think there are some things that we can do to give us a few more spoons over a week. I don't think there is a direct correlation if you eat a banana today, you will be full of energy tomorrow. There are no miracle responses. Just small changes to our way of life that can help (don't worry, I don't manage this every day and often have slip-ups; mostly linked to crisps or takeaways). Use the 80\20 rule, be good 80% of the time and a little naughty the remaining 20%.

I didn't want to accept that I have a set number of spoons and that is 'my lot', I need to find a positive way to look at my life and my restrictions. One day I was discussing old computers and computer games and remembered playing Pac-man when I was younger. I got a fit of giggles, as I thought this game resembled my current situation.

The following is a description of Pac-man from Wikipedia[13]:

"The player controls Pac-Man through a blue maze, eating Pac dots (also called pellets) and fruit. When all Pac-dots are eaten, Pac-Man is taken to the next stage. Four enemies (Blinky, Pinky, Inky and Clyde) roam the maze, trying to catch Pac-Man. Near the corners of the maze are four larger, flashing dots

---

[12] http://www.butyoudontlooksick.com/articles/written-by-christine/the-spoon-theory/

[13] https://en.wikipedia.org/wiki/Pac-Man

known as **power pellets** that provide Pac-Man with the temporary ability to eat the enemies."

I think of my life a little like a Pac-man game. I like to think that if I gobble up fruits, vegetables and healthy food, I'll keep going longer, but I am still chased by the bad guys (symptoms and energy zappers), who can catch me no matter how many vegetables I have eaten. I have identified the Pac man evils for me as follows:

- Blinky: when I am hit by headaches or things that affect my head or eyes
- Pinky: my frequent hot sweats or other issues with my temperature
- Inky: when I get the shakes and other physical symptoms people can see. When they say, 'hey look you are shaking' I am tempted to say, 'do you know, I didn't notice, thanks for pointing that out'. Obviously, I don't, I just smile and say 'it's the drugs'
- Clyde: well, Clyde to me is fatigue, that disruptive character that runs away like Bonny and Clyde but leaves utter destruction behind and I have no control.

When my Pac-man dies, that means I need to sit and rest. When the game ends... I am curled up asleep in bed.

My power pellets are things that give me energy no matter how I am feeling physically, like my children laughing, my husband's cuddles and a Sunday morning spent reading in bed with a cup of coffee. Walking the dog, at whatever speed I can manage helps me to feel brighter, and as though I have achieved something positive. Focusing on the positives help me to feel brighter. All these simple things give me a power pellet. You need to find your power boosts and work out what YOUR healthy foods and actions are. If you can get a few healthy pellets a day and a few power pellets a week you should get a boost. However, remember that even if you have lots of pellets and power pellets, the roaming enemies can still catch up with you. Sometimes there is just no escaping their powers of evil.

I cannot swear to always be doing the right thing for myself; during my first lot of treatment, I put on three stone without caring or even noticing. I started buying larger jeans. The sizes kept creeping up, and I kept telling myself this was just the different sizing in the various shops. It just wasn't important to me at that moment, and when you have the 'dreaded steroids' to blame, you can just keep getting bigger, and nobody says anything. I have old-fashioned scales with a pointer, not a digital reading, and I know if stand on one foot towards the left side I can make that point move at least 2 or 4lbs down. How clever of me, I can pretend I don't have that extra 4lbs even though I know it is there. I've convinced myself that the added weight isn't doing any damage as it is only temporary … it has now been temporary for over 5 years. Maybe it is time to start caring.

Some days weight is genuinely irrelevant for me. Yes, I said it, weight does not matter some days. On other days, when I have caught a glance of my triple chin in a mirror or window, it is soul destroying. My children love to Facetime their dad when he is away with work and one of the hardest things for me is to look at that screen and see the face staring back from the little corner; it isn't me, it isn't the way I think I look. It makes me very sad to see how other people now see me: a pale, overweight, puffed out person. It seems that no matter how much I try and smile, I still look bloody awful, and it feels like the final insult from the illness. I know this sounds very shallow and vain, but it still has a terrible effect on me as it reminds me of what has happened and how my life has changed forever. I think it is more about what it represents inside than how I look externally; it is something that I just cannot hide from people.

It may help some of us to lose those excess pounds, although on some days it really does not matter what you weigh. We live in a world full of perfect images that we cannot help but compare ourselves to; men, women and children. But often the photos are not real. A great example is to look at pictures of the celebrities who go into 'I'm a celebrity get me out of here' and then look at the reality of the same people on camera without the army of make-up artists and creative photography. They are unrecognisable.

My consultant dismisses the weight as a battle for the future and not the present, but I know in my heart that some of my symptoms will ease if I wasn't carrying the excess weight. I think back to Pac-Man and try to remember that the more energy pellets and power pellets I can get the easier it will be to escape the evil enemies. So, my weight battle has become a case of how many healthy things can I eat, and not 'what must I NOT eat'. I find this more natural because it means looking forward to a fresh bowl of strawberries or a spicy bowl of chilli. I still have days where I lose it, but slowly, the weight is shifting, and I feel better for it.

Today I'm having one of 'those days'. I had been feeling great but have had a flare up of the symptoms, and my delightful steroids, aka moon face drugs have been increased 'as a temporary measure' to get things under control. The weight doesn't even come to mind as I sit with a large packet of crisps watching This Morning without really hearing or seeing anything. I know I will regret it in a few days but today that crunch and that mindlessly sitting in front of the TV is helping me; not sure how, but I feel it is. Later I eat a slim fast chocolate bar for lunch. So hilarious, like this will somehow counter the excess.

Some days I am just a daft mindless old bat.

I know my Pac-man idea is right for me: if I eat the right foods for energy and keep moving, I will collect more spoons. So even though I can't do the ideal healthy eating diet every day, I keep trying to do it because if I manage to do it 80% of the time that has got to help me in the battle of the energy zapper.

Please don't misunderstand this chapter. I'm not saying that a healthy diet and a bit of walking will cure you, not at all. Many people have told me over the years, 'oh that's from stress' or 'you should take vitamin x, y or z' or 'why don't you do yoga', or ideas for boosting the immune system (which is strange as it is the immune system doing the damage to me). These things may help how I feel, but they will not cure me, I know this. However, on the flip side, if I don't move out of the house for a week and I order pizza every night, I know that my symptoms, both physical and mental, will get worse.

If we want to battle our illness, we owe it to our bodies to give it the weapons to have a fighting chance in the war. We all know the tools; you cannot avoid health advice, from the news on TV, newspapers or magazines, all offering advice and tips on getting in shape. Please be wary of fad diets though, don't do anything extreme and if you don't know where to start, try searching for 'NHS Diet Advice'. You will find a few websites that can give you reliable and practical advice on losing a few pounds; don't pay out for expensive diets or menus, it can be just common sense. My daughter was given a plate at school that shows what a plate of food should consist of. I think this is all we really need to find healthy meals:

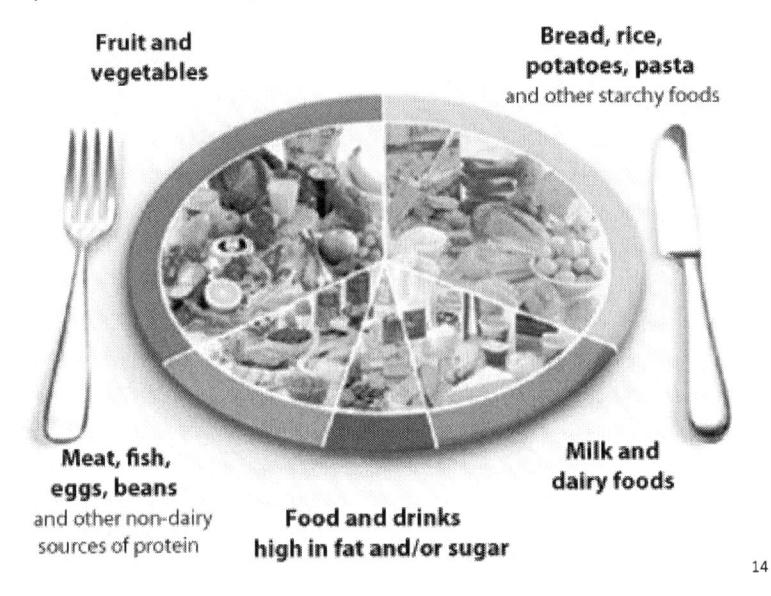

**Fruit and vegetables**

**Bread, rice, potatoes, pasta** and other starchy foods

**Meat, fish, eggs, beans** and other non-dairy sources of protein

**Food and drinks high in fat and/or sugar**

**Milk and dairy foods**

[14]

However, if you do want to track your calories, again don't waste lots of money. I use the free app on my phone called 'My Fitness Pal'. It allows me to search for food and track it daily; it is straightforward, and if you prefer, you can use their website just as easily. With the phone, you can even scan the barcode on the food packet to upload the data. Simple and free. You can even connect it to a fitness tracker, to earn extra calories from doing exercise. I'm sure there are many similar apps or sites for tracking without spending a fortune.

**Obviously, if your doctor has told you not to get moving or to diet, then this isn't an option. But, remember that the eating plate above isn't a diet, it is a healthy balanced meal.**

---

[14] http://www.nhs.uk/Livewell/Goodfood/Pages/the-eatwell-guide.aspx

There are a lot of people in the world who are happy to give you lots of nutritional advice, and often the information or solution will end up costing a small fortune. Be cautious. Dietary advice should be simple, as there is no big complicated message, but the global the weight loss and weight management market is estimated to reach USD 245.51 Billion by 2022 from USD 175.94 Billion in 2017[15]. So, take care not to pay big money; the answer is to eat a varied diet that includes lots of fruit and veg, do a little movement every day, drink lots of water and cut down on alcohol. Oh, and do not smoke! An estimated 89% of lung cancers in the UK are linked to lifestyle factors, including smoking[16].

While having one treatment, I was left exhausted, and I read one of my favourite books ever, Ben Goldacre's Bad Science[17]. I can recommend it as an alternative view of the media push on dietary solutions to every illness. I have found myself falling for many a TV programme showing some miracle cure or the next big superfood, foolish I know. However, sometimes we are just desperate for an easy solution and will jump at any advice given; just be a little careful.

One last piece of advice I was given from a colleague, treat yourself like a car: if you don't put the right fuel in and get it serviced regularly how can you expect it to take you anywhere? And to get the best out of the battery, you need to make sure it goes out for a little drive regularly. We are the same: **we need good fuel, some care and attention and trips out and about to keep everything moving.** As simple as that. Simple but not easy! Keep trying and keep positive.

---

[15] https://www.marketsandmarkets.com/PressReleases/weight-loss-obesity-management.asp

[16] http://www.cancerresearchuk.org/health-professional/cancer-statistics/statistics-by-cancer-type/lung-cancer#heading-Three

[17] http://www.badscience.net/

## Who is your battle with?

Who and what are you really fighting against?

    The illness?

    Yourself?

    The drugs?

    Others who have the same illness?

    Others who have a different illness?

    Other people without a chronic illness?

    Or are you fighting all the above options?

    What value is there in battling any of these things?

    Can you really win any of these battles?

When I first got a diagnosis, my then consultant (he is no longer my consultant), told me I would need three months of treatment and then I would just pop back for a check-up every six months. I left the hospital and felt positive. I thought I could fight and win this battle; I did the inspirational thing and posted on Facebook:

    Bring it on Illness, I will win! The battle starts today.

I got so many likes and positive comments, it was brilliant, we all love a good fight, especially when we can be victorious over an 'evil' illness.

I was very naive and did not understand my illness, or that sometimes doctors don't tell (or maybe they don't understand) the whole truth. I'm learning now. I have a way to go to fully accept the changes this has brought to my life, but I now realise how idealistic and naive I was at the start of this journey. Believing that humans can beat anything. This is human nature, and it is almost like a grieving process of learning to deal with the loss and change you feel in a short period.

Unfortunately, despite the amazing technology available today, we are still helpless against some things.

My fight was not sustainable, and one colleague said:

> 'we are glad you have stopped trying to beat the illness, and you understand you need to sometimes just stop and rest, so you don't look like you are going to collapse on the floor during meetings anymore'.

We can start out fighting, but we cannot sustain it long term. However, we can continue a fight for positivity and acceptance of what our life is going to be in the future. This subtle shift in my attitude does seem to help: switching from fighting the negative to battling to keep positive allows me to find ways to move forward. This is a fight I need to sustain; staying in a positive frame of mind is often difficult because it is very easy to flip into feeling sorry for ourselves, or into believing that our lives are no longer 'worthwhile' because we cannot do everything we used to do. I still have the 'I'm useless' days, and I think that is a normal reaction; my trick now is to try and come back from these days quickly, to allow them to happen but bounce back faster than I did at the beginning of the journey.

The problem with a long-term chronic illness is that it isn't a quick fight, taking a few drugs and having a couple of weeks in bed. It isn't ever an out and out win where the illness is beaten forever. It is a long-term war, with some battles you lose and some you win: It is an on-going campaign. It is a chronic illness, after all.

In the end, the struggle is about getting to a place where you live together, the illness and you, and trying to make the most of the environment you share, making it a positive environment. We all want to rise victorious, maybe carry a flag and wave it triumphantly, but sometimes it is not possible.

I recently watched the astounding Invictus Games[18] ('Invictus' means 'unconquered' in Latin), which are described as:

> "Over 400 competitors from 13 nations will take part in the Invictus Games, an international sporting event for wounded, injured and sick Servicemen and women. Teams will come from the armed forces of nations that have served alongside each other. The Games will use the power of sport to inspire

---

[18] http://invictusgames.org/

recovery, support rehabilitation, and generate a wider understanding and respect of those who serve their country."

It is awe-inspiring to watch: you cry, you cheer, you laugh, you can see the positive effect on those taking part and their families and friends attending. To overcome the physical and mental challenges we face is what makes us human, to beat our disadvantages is humbling and powerful, the Invictus games are a remarkable feat for all involved.

But, I had a sad feeling watching it: I was a little jealous that they could fight; I wanted to follow their lead and get up and take a stand and fight. But I was curled up on the sofa in my pyjamas too exhausted to keep my head up. How could I fight this horrible illness?

I started my battle, telling everybody I will fight and that I will see improvements and my friends will be proud of me and cheer, and I will have life-changing moments of inspiration to post on social media. I wasn't very successful at this fight, there wasn't a way to win. A miraculous recovery was not a possibility.

**It took me a long time to realise my battle isn't one of fighting against the illness; my struggle was to become, in a strange way, a battle with my own self, with my body and my personal ambition. A battle of learning to accept the changes this brought to me, a battle of learning a new language and a struggle to admit that the life I had planned and aimed for was no longer a possibility.**

The life I had planned may no longer be possible, but that's not necessarily a bad thing. My pre-illness life was stressful and filled with work, and my priorities had got a little skewed. I gave so much time and energy to my work; I spent so little time and energy on family or relationships. I wasn't happy, I just pretended I was; I even pretended to myself I was happy (Here I am again lying to myself, but this time it is a little more critical than pretending those extra 4lbs don't exist). Being ill made me look at everything so very differently: I saw my children in a different light, I cuddled them tighter, I understood how distant I had been to my husband and how self-absorbed I had become.

I didn't have a massive change of personality and run off to live in a hippy commune. I didn't take drastic decisions changing my life forever. None of the clichés that appear in Hollywood blockbusters occurred. I will be honest: I did feel a little pressure to… start a charity, raise a million, give up my career and start a dog walking business. But no, I went back to work. Luckily, I had a job that allowed me mostly to work from home, which meant I could carry on, but in a slightly different style. Firstly, I cut right back on travelling: I started to say no to trips and meetings away from home. But I made sure that my work didn't suffer and strangely, I became more productive and focused, and overall, I feel I did my job much better by not running around and spending hours in meetings.

The change in my priorities meant I could have time with my family, but my brain kept on running, and my career path shifted; not a drastic change, just a more realistic version of my future. I know I am lucky that I can work from home, but the world is changing, and this option is open to more people. I remember being at school and being told about 'telecommunication working' as a future possibility and the teacher saying they didn't really think it would ever be possible, but it is. Flexible home working is becoming more and more commonplace and offers those of us who have bodies that cannot keep up with our minds' ambitions a chance to keep working and feeling positive about ourselves.

I have thought long and hard about the fight we have with chronic illnesses; it is a long process, and it can get very dull and tiresome to live with day in and day out. To understand that you have to live with something which affects all parts of your life for the remainder of your life (unless that miracle cure pops up). It is tough to wake up every day and realise that you have this significant impact on your options for the day. I went back to the idea behind the Invictus Games. They stem from an English Victorian poet, William Ernest Henley, who lost a leg due to tuberculosis. He wrote a powerful poem that can really inspire all of us:

Out of the night that covers me,
Black as the pit from pole to pole,
I thank whatever gods may be
For my unconquerable soul.

In the fell clutch of circumstance
I have not winced nor cried aloud.
Under the bludgeonings of chance
My head is bloody, but unbowed.

Beyond this place of wrath and tears
Looms but the Horror of the shade,
And yet the menace of the years
Finds and shall find me unafraid.

It matters not how strait the gate,
How charged with punishments the scroll,
I am the master of my fate,
I am the captain of my soul.

The poem is not only about a physical fight, but also about how we deal with what the world throws at us. My response to whatever is thrown at me is what really matters to my quality of life. For me, the last two lines are what we must embrace.

**I am the master of my fate,**
**I am the captain of my soul.**

I am the master and the captain, I decide my reaction, and I determine my attitude. Today, I choose to be positive and prioritise those things that matter most to me. I may not be able to run a hundred metres, but I can get up and face the world with a smile. That is my way to have an unconquerable soul.

The challenge becomes enormous when you must do this day after day after day, but, we are allowed 'off' days. But we must ensure we get back up and decide our fate, and let our soul sing out to the world. We are often more powerful and resilient than we realise, we need to embrace our strengths.

## Medication

This is a hard one. Read the leaflet in any medication box, there is enough fear there to have you running to throw it in the bin. The list of side-effects and contraindications (this means times when you shouldn't take the medication: for example, you cannot take some medication when you are pregnant, so pregnancy is the contraindication) is often longer than this book. I have a great mix: currently, I am on 22 tablets a day, and this really does get me down. I hate the pills and the biological infusions, I wish I didn't need them, and I hate having to face the reality that I do need them all. The dreaded steroids and the side-effects of my new moon face and rapid weight gain, mixed with mood swings a teenager would be proud off, awful things, all of them.

But hang on, I know that without these little white, yellow and beige pills, I would no longer be alive; **I would not have survived without the medication.**
Maybe I shouldn't hate them so much.

Yes, all medication comes with side effects, just look at a box of Ibuprofen; here is the Ibuprofen side effects list from the NHS website[19]:

> *Ibuprofen can cause a number of side effects.*
> *For this reason, take the lowest possible dose of ibuprofen for the shortest possible time needed to control your symptoms.*
> *Common side effects of ibuprofen include:*
> - *nausea (feeling sick)*
> - *vomiting (being sick)*
> - *diarrhoea (passing loose, watery stools)*

---

[19] http://www.nhs.uk/Conditions/Painkillers-ibuprofen/Pages/Side-effects.aspx

- *indigestion (dyspepsia)*
- *tummy (abdominal) pain*

*Less common side effects include:*
- *headache*
- *dizziness*
- *fluid retention (bloating)*
- *raised blood pressure*
- *gastritis (inflammation of the stomach)*
- *a stomach ulcer*
- *allergic reactions – such as a rash*
- *worsening of asthma symptoms by causing bronchospasm (narrowing of the airways)*
- *kidney failure*

*Less common side effects can also include black stools and blood in your vomit. These side effects can indicate that there is bleeding in your stomach.*

And if this wasn't enough it then adds the following:

*Increased risks*

*Taking ibuprofen, particularly at high doses over long periods of time, can increase your risk of:*
- *stroke – when the blood supply to the brain is disturbed*
- *heart attacks – when the blood supply to the heart is blocked*

*In women, long-term use of ibuprofen might be associated with reduced fertility. This is usually reversible when you stop taking ibuprofen.*

Note: I am not singling out Ibuprofen on purpose, and please don't stop taking them just because of what you read here; if you are worried that you are taking too many, please go and discuss with your GP.

Before I became intimately involved with illness and medication, I would never read these warnings when I was taking tablets for a minor toothache. That is a long list for a pill we can buy over the counter, for a tablet where I can swallow as many as we like for as long as we want. The difference between ibuprofen and my collection of tablets is that I am not forced to take ibuprofen tablets and don't have to schedule them into my daily plans, so I don't resent them; I swallow them willingly and don't think about any damage they may cause me in the future. We don't like to be forced to do something, and when we are angry at being ill or the side-effects of the medication, it is easy to really start to hate those pills.

But surely, hating 'objects' is a bit pointless. They don't care if you hate them; they don't even know you are sending hate messages to them every time you open those little boxes.

Hate is an exhausting emotion and can be all-consuming. It leaves us tired and bitter and angry. I don't know how you feel about this, but I have decided to save that energy and use it more positively. Hating the pills is pointless; they are there to provide us with a better existence. However, if you think that you are getting more negatives than positives from your prescriptions, then maybe they are not the solution for you, and you should discuss this with your doctors. There may be a better solution out there; drugs work differently on different people. Sometimes it is trial and error to find the right combinations for you personally.

Regulators compare the risk to patients from medicine with the benefits the medication will bring them before deciding to approve it for use. This 'Risk vs Benefit' analysis is an objective review of the benefit you can gain compared to the risk of further complications, and the benefits for the patient must outweigh the risks.

Therefore, try and remember that your medication should be bringing you more benefits than risks; it is hard to see the benefits sometimes when you have an extra three stone to carry, or you border on steroid-induced diabetes, or you need a bone density scan to check the medicine hasn't knackered your bones. The benefit is that I am still alive. I am happy to take some risks to get that benefit.

Over time you need to make sure your medication is reviewed by professionals, as improvements in technology and learning are happening all the time. Don't just stay on something for ten years without questioning if it is still the best thing for you. Think of your mobile phone: you check out the upgrades every few years to make sure you are not missing out on something new and helpful. Do the same for your treatment regime.

Steroids are the often most hated medication as their side-effects are so immediate and obvious: mood swings, weight gain, moon face, the list is endless and well known. If you search the internet, you can find many images and horror stories about them. I have been on them for six years now, with the dose ranging from 40mg a day to the fabulous 7mg. I must admit that I haven't managed to stay on 7mg for very long without the illness flaring, and I feel this makes me more than qualified to offer some advice! Yes, they are nasty and have some terrible side-effects, but I also accept that they are miraculous little circles of chalk. When I got the much longed for 7mg a day, I had a flare and struggled to even lift my head. The consultant spoke the dreaded words "we need to increase the steroids"; these six words instantly brought tears to my eyes, as I felt like such a failure. As heart-breaking as this was, within two days of taking 10mg, I felt so much stronger and healthier, just from a couple of extra small tablets a day.

This has now happened many times, and the six words from the doctor still bring tears, but also a strange little relief that I know soon I will feel stronger and able to get some of my positivity back to allow me to keep fighting. I have been told not to take this so emotionally, but I still haven't learnt how to deal with these words calmly, not sure I will ever manage this.

**A few little tips for managing your medication.**

There are ways we can manage our medication to ensure we think about it as little as possible. My GP has an online repeat prescription ordering service that was easy to start using, and it means I don't have to call the doctors' receptionists. I just go online and a few clicks later it is ordered ready for pick up in a couple of days.

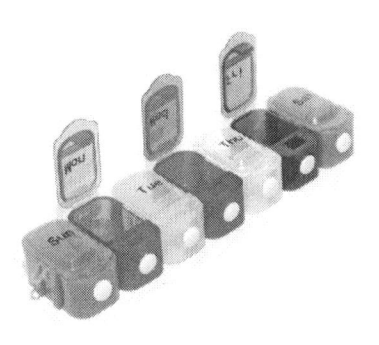

Also, I ask for the prescription to be sent directly to the pharmacy, so I only make one trip. This works great while my medication levels are still changing monthly, as it isn't possible to set up a 'standing order'.

If you have repeating monthly medication, talk to your pharmacy about what repeat prescription services they can offer. Check what 'deals' you can get on your prescriptions, are you eligible for free medication, or can you buy a monthly pass or something similar check here: **https://www.nhs.uk/using-the-nhs/help-with-health-costs/**. Often pharmacies can contact the doctor and get the prescription for you, and all you have to do is go in and pick it up once a month, some pharmacies will even deliver it to you. Work out the best options for you.

One of the main things that really made me feel down was pushing out the pills every morning from their little foil containers; it just reminded me of the number of drugs I needed to take and seeing the warnings each morning reminded me of the severity of the different tablets. I would get the big Tupperware container down and spend a few minutes each day remembering which I needed and how many. This was soul-destroying: a daily reminder of how knackered my body had become. One day while waiting for my bag of drugs at the pharmacy I saw a daily medication box that was multi-coloured and designed so each container could be pulled off and used separately, so if I went away for a night, I could just take one small rectangle instead of a tub of boxes.

I started to 'measure' out my medication every eight days (seven in the little boxes and one lot for the day I do it); this saved a lot of time and emotion. It meant that most days I didn't have to think about the number or severity of the tablets, I could just tip them out and swallow them with a cup of tea in a couple of gulps.

My husband was mean enough to call me an old woman for using the medication boxes, but I have found them invaluable (and they are cheap!). Another advantage I have with these is that my children don't even notice that I am taking tablets anymore as I can do it so quickly. Again, my main aim is to ensure life for them carries on as usual, and watching mum take numerous tablets is not normal.

If you have young children beware, as that they do look a little like toys, so please be careful and ensure they are kept far out of the reach of little hands.

As my pills have now increased and I need different ones in the morning and afternoon, I have purchased a monthly version. So I fill up a couple of weeks at a time; the added advantage of this is that I can see when I am running low on a particular medication and ensure I never run out.

I see comments from people on social media about not taking their tablets or deciding to change their dose without clinical advice. Please don't do this; you increase the risk of unwanted consequences. One of the most significant issues the medical world faces is compliance (i.e. doing as you are told) of taking drugs. You have a prescribed set of medication at a fixed strength as that is what your professional team believe to be the best option for you; if you change or stop the regime, you are entering an unknown and unsupported area. If you don't think your medication is correct or are worried about it in any way, don't stop it; keep taking it and talk to your GP or consultant as soon as you can.

The UK government body, The National Institute for Health and Care Excellence (NICE)[20], states the following about compliance (i.e. taking the medication you have been prescribed in a manner that follows the recommendation):

---

[20] NICE's role is to improve outcomes for people using the NHS and other public health and social care services. We do this by:
- Producing evidence-based guidance and advice for health, public health and

*It is thought that between a third and a half of all medicines prescribed for long-term conditions are not taken as recommended. If the prescription is appropriate, then this may represent a loss to patients, the healthcare system and society. The costs are both personal and economic.*

*Adherence presumes an agreement between prescriber and patient about the prescriber's recommendations. Adherence to medicines is defined as the extent to which the patient's action matches the agreed recommendations.* **Non-adherence may limit the benefits of medicines, resulting in a lack of improvement, or deterioration, in health.** *The economic costs are not limited to wasted medicines but also include the knock-on costs arising from increased demands for healthcare if health deteriorates.*[21]

NICE then talks about two types of non-compliance, intentional and unintentional. Unintentional could be because of a failure to remember, not understanding instructions or physical barriers to taking medicine.

If any of these apply to you or the people you care for then you must discuss options with your doctor; there may be some way, they can help you with the issues faced.

Intentionally not taking your medicines is a different issue and it could be for many reasons: please think about the implications carefully and discuss it honestly with your doctor. I understand that the side-effects are hard to deal with, and we really do need to weigh up the benefits of any treatment compared to the adverse effects we face.

If you feel the life the treatment provides is not the life you want to fight for and the side-effects are too high, then talk to the doctors and your family and friends. Discuss

---

- social care practitioners.
- Developing quality standards and performance metrics for those providing and commissioning health, public health and social care services.
- Providing a range of information services for commissioners, practitioners and managers across the spectrum of health and social care.

[21] https://www.nice.org.uk/guidance/CG76/chapter/ftn.footnote_1

what you can live with and how you achieve that. But please don't just stop the medication! Often drugs need withdrawing slowly, to allow the body to readjust, stopping immediately could cause you serious problems.

If you just decide you don't like taking tablets, maybe think forward about the treatments you may have to confront if you stop taking them. I've faced some horrific things, and now I know that when I put the horrible steroid drops up my nose (as much as I hate that), it is better than the surgery that will be required in the future if I don't do it. So just think about what the long-term future holds for you if you decide not to take your medicines. It is, unfortunately, a balancing game.

## Who to trust with your health?

In the first few years of the illness spent a lot of time waiting: waiting for tests, waiting for appointments, not really feeling that the right things were being done. I wasted a lot of time, a time when my illness was active and attacking me while I sat and waited.

I think the NHS is fantastic, and I trusted that it would work especially hard to ensure I was treated fast and with the best options possible. Again, I was very naive. **The NHS is fantastic**, but it is also enormous (Stats from 2017):

    The NHS deals with around 1.5 million people a day;

    It employs 1.3 million people, that is about, 1 in 23 people in England and Wales;

    GPs see 23 million people each month; and

    An individual GP can see 255 people a week[22].

Suddenly, the individual problems that consume my life, well, don't seem that important. Yet we expect this monster of an organisation to be there for us and solve everything and most of the time it does that, and most of the time it does this just fine.

The NHS is an enormous organisation and has many different sections, which are often run independently and have different rules and regulations, bringing many different challenges. Sometimes things don't pass efficiently between departments. Sometimes not all the 1.3 million people employed by the NHS are entirely dedicated to their job on the day you see them. Sometimes the paperwork does go missing and sometimes … I could go on and on about the issues you could face in getting your right treatment at the right moment.

I am not here to moan about the NHS; I have seen amazing things, and unfortunately, I have seen a few pretty awful things too. My aim here is not to whine or congratulate

---

[22] http://www.nhs.uk/Livewell/nhs-anniversary/Pages/Didyouknow.aspx

the NHS, my purpose is to explain to you that it is **YOUR health and YOUR future you need to concentrate on**.

Ultimately, **you** are responsible for your health, and that involves finding and contacting the best people for you. The NHS can help you, but you need to spend a little time and learn about your condition. This isn't difficult; a quick internet search brings up lots of information. Please only read the information on sites you know, so that could be the NHS Choices website, your individual hospital website or the Mayo, Cleveland clinics' websites in the US. Often each health service or hospital will have information on their website that can direct you to the best place to find facts relevant to you. Patient associations also have an enormous amount of information; find a respected site and read. A 15-minute read could be enough to give you a better idea of your condition, but that could be enough to help you understand what you can do to help improve your situation. Remember Pac-man: little things we do can help improve our overall health. I prefer to print the information out so I can highlight/scribble/re-read the good points over time.

If you want to research more, join social media groups or search for research articles. Research has become much more open in the last few years, and we can often find clinical research information for free. The articles can sometimes be a little overwhelming but remember you don't need to be able to understand everything. You are not reading as a doctor; you are looking for knowledgeable doctors, drug names or treatment options. I read the abstract (intro) and the conclusions first and then skim through the rest for anything interesting, or for similar treatments or symptoms to mine. Look out for the names of hospital consultants referenced, as they may just work near where you live, and you may be able to get transferred to the experts quoted in the research.

If you want to be very thorough, you can set a news alert up on Google for your illness so you will receive an email if it pops up in the news. Remember though that certain newspapers and websites carry stories of miracle cures every day; don't believe everything you read in the newspapers. You can use **https://scholar.google.co.uk/**, https://clinicaltrials.gov/ or https://www.ncbi.nlm.nih.gov/pubmed for searches. You may be a little overwhelmed, but you don't need to read it all, very few people understand the full details of research papers.

**If you can get some background knowledge on your condition and the medication you use, it will give you the understanding and freedom to challenge and discuss what your doctors suggest.** This will help you to have an informed conversation about your future. It is useful to know if your symptoms are common or unusual, you can then query why you still have them. You won't know what is normal for your condition if you don't do that bit of background reading.

We are all terrified of the unknown, and this terror can cause us to panic and worry, and sometimes shout and scream. Once we understand what is happening to us and why, it becomes easier to deal with. I know at some point somebody is going to suggest putting a stent in the large tube that comes out of my heart (the aorta). Initially, this terrified me, but as I have read about it and talked about it, I now keep thinking, 'I wish they would just put the bloody stent in'. **Knowledge is power and power gives us the Invictus Spirit to deal with the situation and fight on. Master and Captain of my soul.**

Different countries have different rules, but in the UK, it is now our right to request to see a specific specialist (search **the internet for NHS Choices**). The NHS constitution states:

> If you need to go to the hospital to see a specialist, you have the right to choose which hospital you're referred to by your GP.
>
> This legal right lets you choose from any hospital offering a suitable treatment that meets NHS standards and costs.
>
> You also have the right to choose which consultant-led team, or a clinically appropriate team led by a named healthcare professional, will be in charge of

your treatment for your first appointment at the hospital. You will be seen by the consultant or by a doctor who works with the consultant in their team.

You have the right to choose where to go for your treatment, but this is useless unless you understand a little about your condition and possible treatment options. You can research hospitals online, and you can contact patient associations to ask for 'centres of excellence'. It may mean travelling a little further for each specialist appointment, but this is your choice, and only you can make it.

My experience was not the best start: I ended up in the A&E ward of my local hospital for several nights, with two different departments trying to deal with me as I didn't fit neatly into one area. After two weeks in the hospital, I was discharged under the care of the renal (kidney) team, I thought this was fine. I had some mild kidney damage, and fluid had built up around the heart, which had been drained by an almighty needle. I was assured the fluid would not return and that the renal team were the best for my illness. I put my faith in the experts.

Initially, I was told I would need high levels of medication for three to six months, and then I would just need check-ups every six months, hence the coming out fighting and thinking I can beat this is three months. Three months came and went, and my drugs were not lowered. Six months came, and I really didn't feel much better, but I was told every month that all my blood tests were coming back healthy, and I was on the mend. Despite a return to the hospital with a nasty chest infection that hadn't been shifted by two lots of antibiotics, nobody seemed concerned that I needed intravenous steroids and antibiotics. I kept on fighting I told the doctors that I couldn't walk upstairs without running out of energy, so I got a chest x-ray, which showed nothing. I was really struggling with lots of vague symptoms (my condition is renowned for this presentation), and yet I came back from each appointment feeling like I had made it up or was just over exaggerating. I was getting down and starting to think I must be imagining my symptoms.

My breaking point came when I received the general clinic follow-up letter, which outlines the appointment discussion and the plans going forward. This is addressed to the GP and copied to the patient. Personally, I think it should be directed to both of us, as this is a little like talking about somebody when they are in the room with you. The inflammatory letter stated "Jane should understand that we all have small things that don't feel right and that she shouldn't expect to find answers to everything. No further tests will be completed, and Jane should consider talking to somebody about her feelings". I was devastated; the letter implied I was making it all up and that if I talked to somebody, I would instantly be cured. As usual, I had a couple of days breakdown to 'process' this latest update.

Then I really came back fighting.

I read the information on my condition, I looked at the patient association material, I looked at which consultants and hospitals were involved in the patient association, I searched research articles and found the writers and where they were based … and I read more. I found that one of the centres of excellence for my rare illness was about one-hour's drive away, and the consultant there seemed to work closely with the patient groups. I decided that as my 'local' hospital was about 25 minutes away, an hour was not too much. I booked an appointment to see my GP to discuss being referred.

The GP meeting was hard, as he had worked with the local renal team for years and thought they were excellent, (which they are for renal problems) but mine wasn't only a renal problem. In the end, I convinced him to write to the centre of excellence, asking for a second opinion. I got the appointment through before I was due to go back to the renal team, so I cancelled my appointment at the local hospital and never went back there. This was my best decision ever and probably saved my life.

The first day of the new hospital was terrifying, so many different emotions: what if I had made a mistake and I was just pathetic, what if the hospital agreed with the old hospital and told me to just get on with it? Millions of thoughts swamped my head. At my first appointment, I saw the big boss and his first question was, 'why do you want a second opinion?' I don't think I had expected such a direct question. I remember looking at him, feeling like I had been sent to the headmaster and just saying, 'I know I am not improving on the medication, but my current doctors don't seem to believe me'. He didn't comment or say anything negative; he just reviewed all my version of my history.

**One thing that proved very useful was that I had kept all my paperwork: the biopsy results, the clinic letters, appointment letters for tests, the discharge notes from hospital stays. They were all in chronological order and therefore gave the perfect summary of my history. A good tip: a little bit of organising your paperwork can save you long conversations and questions.**

Another thing I have learnt is that doctors can speed read these letters and just miss out the polite bits; just take in the facts very quickly. Remember to keep all the relevant paperwork. Create a file; this will allow you to reference information accurately and rapidly. I carry a folder with the last six months information and file the rest at home. However, for any big review meeting, I bring essential documents from the previous few years ... better to be prepared (do not keep everything, try and work out what is necessary).

To this day, I think this was one of the most challenging meetings of my life. So many emotions and so much at stake. But in the end, it was so gratifying when this senior expert said, 'Yes, I think your illness is still active, and I will take over your treatment'. Pure relief.

When you get an expert, they know what to look for, and all of a sudden, my discussions with doctors were based on facts and some serious tests. I was given MRIs and CT scans, and they did identify evidence of severe, active illness; an active illness that supported my symptoms and showed an urgent, life-threatening issue. The liberation you feel when you can point to a reason why you feel so terrible rather than somebody writing that maybe you should 'talk with somebody' is indescribable. I was vindicated for requesting my change in hospital.

My horror returned when I realised how few of my friends knew that you could request to see a different consultant or hospital as part of your rights within the NHS constitution; friends said to me 'you are so lucky that you knew what to do'. I hadn't known I could do this either; for me, it came from the desperation of not being believed by my team of professionals. Currently, I have a tremendous specialised team who work hard to make sure I am seen by any additional specialists as my illness is a systemic illness, which means it affects multiple organs or the whole body. Looking at just my renal organs was never going to help me recover.

The NHS is awesome and powerful and works miracles, but it is not ultimately responsible for your health; **you are.** So, do your research, read a little, talk to your GP and patient associations, join social media groups and watch what people say. Then make the right choice for you and, if somebody questions your rights to choose, go to the NHS website, print out the NHS constitution, take it in and show them that you do have the choice. I firmly believe that the NHS saved my life, but I also think that if I hadn't exercised my option within the NHS, I might not be here to write this.

So, care about yourself and take some time to think about your options.

**GP receptionists**

I'm not sure how to start talking about this, I have heard such horror stories about dealing with the reception team at GP surgeries, and I have had a few minor run-ins over the years. However, generally, I find if you are **very polite** and nice, you can seem to get them to understand you and your issues. My politeness is almost too over the top, but it does seem to work well, I also highlight that I have a long-term disease, and I am immune suppressed in the first few words. I think that when you highlight your situation early on it places emphasis on them to try and help you. Having said that I do remember a day when my daughter had banged her head at nursery quite severely, and

I turned up at the GP's at 6.01, and they wouldn't let me see a doctor or nurse as they shut at 6pm. I was not amused when I then had to sit in A&E for four hours to be seen and it turned out to fine. So, try and stay calm, factual and highlight what you need and any extra critical information you need to share, and cross your fingers that they are in a good mood.

## Clinical trials

Clinical trials happen across all areas of health, and most will bring benefit to future sufferers of your illness. You may be asked to take part in one during your journey, but please remember that you are under no obligation to participate in any clinical trial. I have been involved in a number (I think this is because I have a rare illness); some have only required me to complete a form, others have involved blood samples being taken and the main one involved me trialling a 'biological' treatment via infusions.

For each trial, I trusted my doctor to suggest only the beneficial trials, and I read the material and did a little research. I agreed only after I had done my own background checks. I have been lucky in that my doctors keep me updated on the progress of trials and I can also check them via a website, where I can view newsletters and the material given to all involved in the trial (this was for the main one I was involved in). So I feel that, although the treatment didn't work that well for me, I know there was knowledge gained from what I shared. If you want to read the details of any clinical trials, they should be registered on the website: **www.clinicaltrials.gov**.

When you are asked to participate in a clinical trial, you may want to help others, and most of us think we should help, but you need to take control of your treatment and your future life. Therefore, if you are asked to participate in a clinical trial, you should not feel you have to be included, and if you feel pressure to be involved you should make a complaint against the person applying the pressure; it is your choice. It may sound selfish and cruel, but you must be convinced the trial is worth any increased risk you will face. Talk it through with the doctor, ask for as much information as you feel you want to see, there are no silly questions when it comes to your health, get all the facts, risks, benefits. You can also ask who is funding the trial.

You are also within your rights to ask who is funding the trial and if the results are shared with you. Clinical trials are often financed by the manufacturers of the products (Drug or Medical Device) under test. You may wish to ask about the implication of a negative result from the trial: how will these benefit future generations? Will these results also be shared? If you are providing time, effort, personal information, blood, and other samples, and you are increasing your risk, you have a right to ask any questions you think appropriate. If you don't get the answers, then you can make the decision on the lack of information you get.

**Participation in clinical trials is your decision, and you should be comfortable that it is right for you. Do not feel pressure to be involved.**

Never make the decision on the spot. Take a little time to think about it, speak to your GP, who should be on your side and impartial about the success of the trial. It is great to think that we could help others, but just consider what the additional risk is for you. Then weigh up your options carefully.

### What if you have a reaction to your treatment?

If you have an adverse reaction to treatment or medication, you should see your doctor, but you should also notify the right association to ensure that they can monitor all the similar effects that are occurring. I don't think many people know about this option and it indeed isn't an immediate thought if something doesn't go according to plan. As with clinical trials, we naturally want to help others, and generally, we do not want to say bad things about drugs or devices that we rely on for our health. Think of the situation in a slightly different way: we jump to participate in clinical trials, but we shy away from feeding back the negatives of our treatment. However, by not feeding back the negatives, we are allowing others to experience the same bad side-effects.

Each country or cluster of nations has a process for collating this feedback. In Europe, each country should share with the rest of Europe so that any trends or serious side-effects can be identified very quickly. The analysis of negative reactions can only occur if we, the users, feed the details back to the regulators; otherwise, they will never know. If you experience an unexpected side-effect, first seek treatment and advice from your doctor and then ask if they will be reporting this to the relevant body; if not, then you must report this issue.

In the UK, the government regulator is the Medicines and Healthcare products Regulatory Agency (MHRA). It runs the side-effects reporting scheme and if you search Google for 'MHRA Yellow Card' or 'MHRA side effects' you will find the correct webpage. MHRA describes the system as follows:

> The Yellow Card Scheme is vital in helping the MHRA monitor the safety of all healthcare products in the UK to ensure they are acceptably safe for patients and those that use them. Reports can be made for all medicines including vaccines, blood factors and immunoglobulins, herbal medicines and homoeopathic remedies, and all medical devices available on the UK market.
>
> The Scheme collects information on suspected problems or incidents involving
>
> - side effects (also known as adverse drug reactions or ADRs)
> - medical device adverse incidents
> - defective medicines (those that are not of acceptable quality)
> - counterfeit or fake medicines or medical devices
>
> It is essential for people to report problems experienced with medication or medical devices as these are used to identify issues which might not have

been previously known about. The MHRA will review the product if necessary, and take action to minimise risk and maximise the benefit to the patients. The MHRA is also able to investigate counterfeit or fake medicines or devices and if necessary, take action to protect public health.

FDA (Food and Drug Administration) in the USA also runs a similar scheme. If you search 'FDA Med Watch', you will see similar information to the above and a straightforward way to report issues. For all other countries, I would just search for your country name and 'patient adverse reaction'. Manufacturers also run studies after products are placed on the market called 'post-market surveillance' studies. In theory, these should ask proactively for feedback, but I have NEVER been asked for feedback on any of the products I have been given. So I believe that as patients, we should be proactive and feedback on any issues we face.

## Cheese sandwich again?

"Girls, cheese and cucumber sandwich with crisps - go wash your hands."

"Woohoo, can we have monster munch?"

So easily pleased, my two beautiful young girls. As happy as they are to have the fake taste of pickled onion, I wonder where my spice has gone, where has my excitement gone? This must be the third night this week I've given them cheese sandwiches. Really, is that as good as I can do?

Can I just point out that they had a hot school lunch each day, so I wasn't depriving them of anything, I had just lost my zest and enthusiasm for life completely. Dealing with an illness that never stops is draining and trying to conserve your energy, for minimal reward, day after day is very tedious.

Life becomes dull, safe and just mind-numbingly functional.

I managed to get through the days and keep everything afloat, but I lost a considerable amount of the exuberance I had for life; life became very flat. The most exciting thing seemed to be treating myself to a cappuccino on my own, as I was too tired to talk to people. This became the most pleasurable moment of my week. Yet a lonely cappuccino is just some milk and coffee in a place that isn't as nice as my own front room.

When your whole-body aches or you feel too tired to get dressed, it is hard to make time for enjoyment; but there is also the feeling that if you have some fun and laugh, people may not believe that you really are ill. I regularly faced the clichéd comments of 'well you don't look sick', or 'give yourself time, it will all sort itself out', or 'I have to take tablets too, you just have to get on with it'. These comments have all come from friends and some also from healthcare professionals. They are meant to cheer you up, but really, they just make you feel more pathetic. They make you think the person does not really believe that you have a serious ongoing illness. So, when faced with these 'kind' comments, you do feel guilty about going out and having a giggle. I try (I don't always succeed) to ignore the comments and take them in the manner they are meant. I think the meaning is really something like, 'I'm not sure what to say to you, and I so want to make you feel better, so I'm going to say something positive to try and help'. When you think of the comments in this way, they are kind-hearted but a little misguided.

Enjoyment and pleasure are essential, and they are not out of bounds. If you had broken your leg, you would not be worried about letting somebody see you laugh or try to walk, it is not an issue when you have physical proof of your pain. When the pain is hidden, we feel we need to show it externally to be believed. I have done this a lot and, as I write this sentence, I really wonder why I do this. When I had a toothache, I went to extraordinary lengths to NOT show how much pain I was in, yet here I am during chemotherapy feeling that I have to tell or show physical symptoms of pain to any friend that talks to me. I feel guilty if I put full makeup on and do my hair because admittedly, I am too sick to care about my appearance. The chemo has left me very pale with some monster bags under my eyes, and my gut reaction is to let this all show on the school pick up so that everybody can see the pain and discomfort I am in. This is utter crap. Crap crap crap. Yet I still do it.

What a mixed message I am giving to myself and others: I don't want to talk about my illness and my terrible struggle, but here I am trying to show the world how awful I can look. Writing this is like a light bulb going on, my own little eureka moment. I hadn't realised that I had actually been aiming for sympathy and questions. I had been waiting for anybody to notice me and ask if I am ok so I can hint at how hard it has been for me and what a martyr I am for keeping going - all for the sake of my kids, of course. Wow, I have become the person I am trying to say you must not become. It is simple for life to become just about the illness, to be able to change all conversations back to how awful your life has become since diagnosis.

How dull I have become?

Am I a cheese sandwich when I used to be a chilli infused fondue?

**How do you escape the dull and get back to some spice?**

Firstly, cheese sandwiches can be good wholesome food and some days we just need a cheese sandwich, but we also need something to set our senses alive. Having lost significant taste and smell during treatment, I can confirm that bland is boring. However, igniting our senses takes effort and imagination, and I believe this is where the issue lies. When you are tired, and your thoughts are dulled by the daily concoction of drugs, it is difficult to conjure up imagination; even if you can imagine something unusual, the effort required to organise this can be more than we can face taking on.

So, having realised that I have become all about my illness and that I have lost my 'spunk', as my years of watching Neighbours as a child taught me, it is now time to change this. To get some spark back, I have set some simple challenges aimed to get my spunk back. If you are reading this and feeling that maybe your life has gone off the boil a little and you are not ready for life to be lukewarm, then join me to tackle a few of the ideas and see how you get on. Here is my initial list of fun things:

- **Bake proper garlic bread**. Search Google for Paul Hollywood Garlic Bread, I promise it was terrific. I will be making this again soon.

- A trip to the **Children's Farm**, followed by **Sunday lunch** out, fun followed by food and no washing up to finish.

- As a family **make mozzarella cheese** and use it to make individual homemade pizzas. My husband made the pizza bases; we all helped make the sauce and the cheese, and then created our own pizzas. A great family experience. The pizzas tasted tremendous and making the cheese was entertaining. I bought the kit on Amazon, but you do need a lot of milk!

- Turn the radio on and sit down with an **'adult colouring book'**. This is a new phenomenon which had completely passed me by, but my old friend had sent me one during my treatment and urged me to have a go. I had put it on the side and giggled about it. It is based on art therapy, which uses different parts of the brain, and I admit I was sceptical. After an hour of colouring, I was smiling and looking at a beautiful image; the hour passed quickly, and the smile lasted throughout the day. I really did enjoy this and will do it again. Thank you, Alex, and I apologise for doubting your wisdom.

- Construct a **Gingerbread house** (you can buy kits). Not sure it tasted great, but it took us back to the fun childhood story. This prompted a bedroom search for the book, which we then read together.

- Buy a **new book**, something you don't typically read, and sit and read it for at least two hours without moving (toilet and tea stop's allowed). I chose Kate Adie's Biography; I can recommend it.

- Meet a friend at a **Forestry Commission Woodland** and go for a gentle 30-minute walk. She described my walking as snail's pace, but I thought it was perfect for watching the world go by. The coffee shop at the end was wonderful.

- Think about some of the lovely people who have stuck with you and **write short letters** to them; not a huge essay, just a simple thank you for being your friend.

- Have a go at tidying your **garden.** I know this may not sound fun, but the sense of achievement I felt when I did it was immeasurable. As I sat looking out of my window, I was tired but so happy to have pushed myself.

- Feeling a bit stiff and tired? Finish reading your book, have a long **bath and put a facemask on**.

- Enjoyed the fresh air: drive to **a country park** (for me it was Burghley Park in Lincolnshire) and go for another gentle walk in the grounds. I did this on my own, and it was amazing to see how beautiful the gardens were at my own pace.

- Join a friend at a yoga class. Mine was described as **'restorative yoga'** and was very slow and gentle, but I could feel some huge stretching going on. Afterwards, I felt brilliant.

- Get your **nails** painted and have a pedicure (maybe not a man-thing!). I did it to try and sort out the horrible skin on my feet, which have appeared since my diagnosis, seeing the improvement made me smile, lots.

- Take your little one to a **disco party** and let yourself go on the dance floor (yes, I know: embarrassing mum). I only lasted a few minutes, but it was such fun, or if you don't have kids, just go dancing.

- Take the children **roller skating.** I was terrible! (again, go without kids)

- Have a gadget-free rest day. The kids were back at school, so I decided to use **no electronic gadgets** all day: phone, TV, tablet and computers all off. Not sure the house has ever been so clean, and I'm not sure I recommend it either!

- Buy yourself a bunch of **flowers**! Go on, you deserve it.

- **Write a poem**. Mine will never be shared in public.

- Spend time reading the **Make-a-Wish** website. In between crying, I donated to help make a wish come true. It really can help to put things into perspective.

- **Invite friends for Coffee and cake** at your house, to thank people who have been amazing.

- Go **wine tasting** at the local wine shop. It was such fun … may have bought a bottle too many.

- Have a 'Movie Day' and make **homemade popcorn.** We stayed in PJs.

- **Go on a picnic** (cheese sandwiches allowed). We went to the 'lake beach' at Rutland water: pork pie, crisps, sandwiches and a few silly games. Just perfect.

- **Have a 'Formal Family Meal'.** We all got dressed up smart, and I cooked a three-course meal. Who needs restaurants?

- Have a relaxing **facial.** Peaceful, resting, and my one smelt of beautiful roses.

- **Breakfast** out at the garden centre and then pick your favourite flowers, bring them home and plant them (you can get the family to plant them for you).

- Buy a **trashy magazine** and read (although there isn't much to digest) all the gossip. It did make me giggle, but I don't think I will repeat this one too often; I think I felt more depressed by the end of it. Apparently, my hair, figure, romance and job aren't 'perfect' enough for the fantasy world these magazines aim to show you.

- **Make a photo album**. We picked our favourite pictures from the year, put them into an online album and sent it to print.

- **Have a 'Date Night'** with your husband or significant other. We had tuna steak and fries, cheesecake and a little wine.

The list just gave me a little push and made me smile. **It is easy to get stuck at 'being ill', but with a bit of effort, you can add some meaning to the days. You don't have to go off climbing a mountain or run a marathon to show that you are fighting and that you will not be beaten by your illness.** The activities with the kids taught them that I am still fun even if I cannot do all the things, I used to be able to do, and it really gave us a good laugh to do things together.

Thinking up the ideas has brought a bit more zest into my life and made me realise that if I get up off my butt and move or try something new, I have more energy than I thought. Granted, some of the activities required me to retire to bed for an hour to recuperate, but they were worth it.

If you struggle with ideas, search for bucket list ideas on the internet, and you will have more ideas than you can cope with. I have created a longer-term bucket list that isn't right for this book, but I will be working hard at ticking off things from the list - including the exciting plan of going off to soak in the Blue Lagoon in Iceland (I need to start saving up my pennies).

## Remission, relapse are just words

There are so many emotional words to do with illnesses; some people still like to whisper some of them, to make them less real. I remember so clearly a comedy sketch where the mother couldn't mention the word 'cancer' without whispering it. At the time I found it funny, partly because the world was different a few years ago but also because it was true; when we are uncomfortable or nervous, we react in strange ways. Some people will whisper, some will screech words and others will try everything possible to avoid words. People react to medical terms in very different ways, and this applies both to those of us who suffer and those who try and support us. Understanding this discomfort around the words themselves can help us reflect upon the reactions the words elicit from hearing them.

In our world of social media and PR, some illnesses have become something of cartoon baddies: something we need to 'come and get', something that we must fight and that we get called brave for fighting. I understand the logic, but what happens when you don't feel brave, or you know you are losing the fight? Does this add an extra burden to our guilt at not winning or letting others down? Does it make you a better person if you fight valiantly against being ill?

Illness is not a comedy monster we can hit with a rubber sword. Don't get me wrong, I agree we need to fight against it and learn how it works to try and defeat it, but I don't think we should be humanising it and making it a personal fight against a demon.

I spoke earlier about my nervousness around the PR of illnesses and having patient associations fighting each other for awareness and funding. It leads to the most high-profile diseases getting most of the support. This is not how I feel the world of healthcare should get funding, but I think we have gone past the point of reverting back. It is no longer impressive to run a marathon to raise money – that's been done many times – now you must run 100km or do 10 marathons over 10 days. Whatever next? Maybe a charity supporting those damaged during extreme fundraising events?

Research is needed into all illnesses, and the funding per illness shouldn't be based on the use of emotional language; it should be based around facts, that are compiled and reviewed by clinicians, scientists and experts; not reviewed by journalists, marketing teams or the loudest fundraisers. The fact that at the start of my illness, several people said, 'well at least it isn't cancer', shows how one illness has been elevated above all others. The comments from friends made me feel like I didn't have a proper illness because it wasn't labelled as cancer.

**Names of medicines**

I have faced a lot of new words in my journey, most of them I wished I had never had to learn.  Just getting your head around some of the drug names is challenging enough, but it's when the words take on an added meaning that the emotional side becomes involved.  I have swallowed and been injected with many drugs over the last few years; all have a job to do, all have side effects, and I would prefer not to take any of them. But three of these have stood out in my mind and have taken on a strangely personal part of my life.  They can be called the Good, the Bad and the Ugly:

- Thyroxin (the Good):  This is to correct my faulty thyroid, which makes me sleepy. I know there are side-effects to this drug, but I cannot tell you what they are because it never bothered me, so I never looked them up.  All I thought about was that my thyroid could be the cause of my energy loss and weight gain… once this drug kicks in I will be a Size 8 triathlete (I'm not and probably never will be, even though my thyroid is now medically under control).  I am so blinded by the fact that this drug may help me lose weight; I do not consider there may be any negatives.

    How very shallow of me to just think about the weight aspects?  I didn't consider the side-effects of the treatment; I don't think I ever thought about the seriousness of my thyroid not working correctly as it was not my primary illness. It was a consequence of other issues and never the central focus for me. I saw the outcome of taking the tablets as only positive. Whereas for my 'main illness' I joined the patient association and the social media page, for my thyroid illness, I just carried on with no support and minimal knowledge. I think this attitude comes from considering the treatment as positive; I had no issue with taking it or increasing the dose (in my mind increasing the dose meant more weight loss). I am a little embarrassed by my naiveté. For information, because of all the other things going on in my body, I have never lost weight due to the thyroxin!

- Cyclophosphamide (the Bad): I spent a long time trying to avoid this treatment, but it caught up with me, and I had to undergo the dreaded 'Chemo'. This involved sitting in a hospital chair for 6-7 hours while the infusion dropped into my body. Cyclophosphamide is a well-used and trusted chemotherapy agent, with years of clinical use and some horrific side-effects. My first experience was not good: I remember suddenly needing to go to bed and trying to crawl up the stairs while thinking I may just be sick down the stairs. Truly horrendous for me, and for my husband who had to watch this and then tuck me up in bed as I was crying. But the emotional aspect of this drug does not come from the side-effects; it comes from the fact that when you tell people you are starting chemo, you get an instant outpouring of kindness, sympathy and love. It's almost like the world thinks this is the worst thing you can ever face and, I think this is because they can understand some of what will happen to you, it makes it easier to empathise. Having an illness or a treatment that people recognise and can understand, allows people to sympathise and easily support you. When something is entirely alien, and they have no understanding, people do not know what to say to you or how to support you in your journey. I understand this and would probably be the same before my own horrible experience.

I had a long journey before chemo and had many nasty side-effects from drugs, but it was difficult for friends to understand these as I didn't want to share full details and the media are not that interested in those treatments. The word chemo is emotional, and I discovered that for most people, the first question was about my hair. I do admit to feeling a little like a fraud when I only had a bit of thinning hair and that, because I had so much to start with, nobody could tell I had lost any. I am convinced that some people thought that the lack of hair loss meant I couldn't be having any other 'typical' side-effects. I can assure you that just because somebody does not lose their hair, it does not indicate that they have a smooth ride! I hid so much and left the smile on my face to prevent questions, the sickness was uncontrollable…but I turned up to the school gate, smiling.

This drug has saved my life, but it also puts my life at risk in both the medium and long-term and that is something I have to accept and live with. I don't hate this treatment, which I think is because in this case, we expect the side-effects, as they are discussed so publically, and we all know somebody who has had to face them.

However the word Chemotherapy is one of the most emotional words in the world, so to limit the reaction I would get I nearly always started the sentence with, 'it's not given in the same way as for cancer'. I thought this would help keep people calm, but I think the only thing it did was to make people believe I wasn't suffering from the treatment. I should never have used this phrase; it undermined everything I went through.

- Prednisolone/Steroids (the Ugly): if you search for this medicine on Google and look at the image tab, you will see lots of memes of what this drug does to you. My personal favourite is the hamster cheek phenomenon, which I have now personally suffered from for about six years. I think my face is at least a third wider than it used to be before steroids. I have had so many 'kind' comments about the weight gain and hamster cheek side effect: 'you have a lovely round face normally, so you still look great'; 'we know it isn't you, it's the drugs that cause the weight'; 'it will go soon'; 'you still look pretty'; and the best, 'we still love you'. While these, absolutely have been said with kindness, when you look in the mirror and see something that horrifies you, these comments don't really bring any comfort.

Prednisolone, like other steroids, has other less obvious but still common side-effects, such as lack of sleep, mood swings, shaking, reduced bone density, increased risks to cancers and many more. The loss of sleep makes everything else seem ten times worse, and the shaking just highlights to everybody that you have a problem. I used to see my family watching my hands, trying to see if they were shaking. They did it out of concern, but it made me feel dreadful that they could observe the effects I was feeling. My nine-year-old used to shout out, 'Mummy you are shaking, sit down and rest!'; this broke my heart every time.

All of this and more make Prednisolone or Steroid the most emotional words I have heard in my journey, but it is a fantastic drug that is used in so many ways and has such amazing results. The positive effects I get from it are far higher than any other medication I have taken, but yet I still hate it; I hate that as soon as it is increased my knees swell to double the size. Emotional is not a strong enough word for this tablet, but in all the searches regarding it, you never really see the words that should be used: **essential to keep so many people alive, a real wonder drug**.

So these are my good, bad and ugly of the treatment world. Emotionally I feel very different about these three drugs. When I write it down, it really does seem a shallow review of the three, because without them I would not be alive, and yet I feel so differently about them all. I wonder how I would feel about each of them if I'd been given them without being told of the side-effects and I didn't know what they were called.

**Remission**

Throughout a journey with any illness, we go through phases. I talked about my journey earlier in the book, where I explained how desperate I was to beat the illness and get the magic comment from the doctor that I was in remission. I don't think desperate is a strong enough word for how much I wanted to hear the word remission. Frantic may be more appropriate, but even this doesn't adequately express the desire I felt to reach this 'nirvana' like state.

My lack of understanding was apparent; remission is not always a single point in the journey, it is not that one day when I would wake up and be in remission, not for me anyway. I had put so much emphasis on this nirvana state that I wanted to put everything on hold until I reached the magic day when I could say I was in remission. Unfortunately, I haven't managed to stay in a meaningful remission for more than six months in the last six years.

**What a waste of time waiting for a magic word to be said. I should have just been living for the moment and enjoying everything I could. Back to my favourite quote from Buddha; it is tough to do, but I keep trying: "Do not dwell in the past, do not dream of the future, concentrate the mind on the present moment."**

If we always want to go back to our old self or dream of a future where we will be 'well', we miss all the fun now. I missed a lot of fun, but now I try not to miss anything. Even if it means my husband running around trying to find a seat for me at a friend's birthday so I will not be stood up for too long, or everybody making sure I drink lots of water if I have a glass of champagne. Or that I sit down when I am at the park with the kids and then occasionally go down the slide like a woman possessed. **Keep the Invictus Spirit and wake up each day with a little fight in you that says, 'today will be the best day I can make of it.'**

Doctors need to track the progression of our illness, they need to see if the medication is working, they need to monitor our side-effects, and they need to declare if an illness is in remission. However, this declaration may not signify a significant change for us as patients. It may mean that we have things under control or that we are clear of active illness; it does not always mean that we are back to how we were before the illness appeared.

This was my colossal misunderstanding: I thought if I reached remission, I would be back to 100% health. But illnesses leave behind consequences of their actions, which depends on the illness and its severity, so please don't assume that when a doctor talks about remission they mean that you will be back to normal health. Remission may not mean that you are the same as you were at the start of your journey.

You need to take control of all these emotional words and think logically. Ask the doctors what remission means FOR YOU, or what the treatment will DO TO YOU; don't believe that because something is a familiar word that you don't need to have a full understanding of what it will mean TO YOU. Remission will mean different things to different people.

Ask questions. Write the items out before you see the doctors, write down the answers (or record the conversation, most doctors are happy for you to record the discussion). Research your condition on reliable websites. Don't just google random websites, you could be reading from a totally crazy site with no scientific basis whatsoever. Be sure you take time to think about the words associated with your illness, do you understand what they mean FOR YOU?

Do the words cause you to react differently? Does it really matter?

Maybe you are desperately trying to reduce your steroids but happy to increase the thyroxin, or perhaps you have your life on hold for remission.

Only you know the answers to these questions, so you need to be honest with yourself.

**Above all, please ask what the words really mean FOR YOU and YOUR LIFE.**

## Inspiring? Me?

Inspiring? Several years ago, a passing comment from a friend made me think about this word and how it applies to life with an illness. We all see the stories, the awards ceremonies and the tear-jerking TV interviews. We have a perfect stereotype of people, for somebody fighting an illness, we see a brave person battling, staying strong and trying to put on a smile. Not sure that is what my friend meant, it was more about the fact that I got out of bed each morning and smiled on most of those days. These stereotypes pile on the pressure to be 'perfect' and face the world in the 'expected' way.

So, am I inspiring? On the outside maybe, but not to those closest to me... probably more like moaning and negative!

I don't feel inspirational to myself, and I doubt my close family think I am either.

I am not sure I am searching for praise, more like trying to avoid discussions around the whole illness thing. Yet somehow, I am told I am inspiring. I find this totally bizarre; the last thing I feel is that I am inspiring to anybody. The Oxford English Dictionary defines inspire:

> Fill (someone) with the urge or ability to do or feel something

I don't think I have filled anybody with any kind of urges for a long time. But I just keep going, whatever happens. I feel more like Dory in 'Finding Nemo' where she sings 'just keep swimming, just keep swimming'. I just keep going, trying to maintain some sort of normality, with the strange hope that one day I will attain real normalcy.

**My main thoughts always are to keep it as normal as possible and to make that appear effortless. And yes, this does leave me feeling deflated and exhausted a fair amount of the time. It is my choice, and I stand by the fact that I have people who rely on me; I love them so much that I put all my effort into making their world seem stable and normal. Stable and normal can verge on impossible and boring, but I hope**

**that by keeping the world steady, my family will see only limited effects from this dreadful illness.**

As with everything I have written, this doesn't always work. There are moments when I scream and shout and give in like we all do, illness or not. Initially, I was hard on myself and berated myself over these slips, but over time, I have realised that they are standard for everybody. Just because my children must face living with a sick mother doesn't mean they always need to see a perfect mother. The world isn't perfect, and they need to grow up knowing this. None of us is perfect all the time, but I think that when we have a chronic illness, we seem to feel that any loss of composure is down to the illness. I confess to wondering if some of my grumpiness is just down to getting older. For example, is the slight reduction in my eyesight because of the steroids or the natural decline that comes from entering into my 40s? It is easier to blame the 'damn steroids', but I suspect age plays a large part in this change, the problem is that I no longer understand what my body should be like at this age without an illness.

So, if people expect you to be inspirational, what does this look like? I felt pressure to start a patient charity, but there was already a great one available; no point in competing with a great charity, raise millions of pounds and spread the word to anybody who would listen.

Instead, I did a few simple things: I set a standing order up to the charity that had helped me, I shared a few web links on my Facebook page. I completed a 24-hour sponsored silence (I was too tired to do anything more exciting, but it did raise nearly a thousand pounds, which shows you how much I like talking and how much people would pay to shut me up). None of this changed the world or meant Hollywood wrote a film about me; does this mean I failed?

I don't think I failed in being ill, I just didn't believe all the hype that is created in the media about how this should be a catalyst to great things. The media enjoy an exceptional story and only cover events that are out of the ordinary. Because they include so many of these, we start to believe that these 'unusual stories' must be 'the normal', and we are quick to compare ourselves to them.

An everyday example of this is seen in how the media covers parenthood and giving birth. Apparently, according to many a celebrity (often selling a book or a new baby product they designed), giving birth is the most magical and life expanding experience of their life. They find being a mother a wonderful experience that cannot be compared, all the time running around with the kids means they are instantaneously able to do another swimwear photo shoot two weeks after giving birth. As a woman who really struggled for the first few months (probably years) after giving birth, I hated these women for making me feel like a failure in what should have been a relaxed, non-judgemental time in my life. Some days I didn't manage to get out of my smelly pyjamas, which I had been living in for the previous two weeks (I do not think I am the only mother to do this regularly).

These celebrities did not inspire me. And I think over time after a few have confessed to having postnatal depression and feeling enormous pressure to appear perfect, I feel very sorry for them. And yet more of these 'wonder-mums' pop up each year. Please stop, just be an ordinary mum and show your faults. The same occurs will illness, we look around for inspiration of how to cope with this new world, and it can be tough to find a real story without the media slant of a hero or horror stories. When a story is featured in the media, it is only a snapshot of somebody's life, it does not show the years before or after, which may have been full of boring days.

**Inspiring does not come from being perfect. Inspiring comes from your response to what life throws at you and how you deal with the fallout. You are reading this because you have a chronic illness (or maybe you care for somebody with one). This is what life has thrown at you; you cannot change it, and there is little point in wondering 'why me?' Your decisions in life, focus on how you, as an individual deal with the illness going forward.** There is a lot of scientific research that shows significant links between remaining positive and feeling healthier. However, when a doctor dared to mention this to me, I thought he was implying that my illness was all in my brain. How dare he? Yet, over time, I have realised what this means, and it is nothing to do with making your illness up.

One of my main struggles was around being told things I wasn't allowed to do anymore. I was told that I would never be able to go for a run again by one doctor. This made me cry and feel destroyed for a few days. Then I decided this would be the thing on which I would prove the doctors wrong, this would be my 'inspiring story' of how I overcame my illness to win the London marathon! So I decided my test of feeling better would be to run another half marathon; I dreamt about it.

Six years later and I still cannot run, but I don't cry about it anymore. I decided that the objective of 'running again' was actually leaving me more stressed and upset than anything, it was not a safe objective for me to pursue. So I changed my objective to something a little more realistic: I walk for 30-60 minutes a day. This means that I hit my 10,000 steps a day and my legs are looking better than they have for years, but I'm not putting any pressure on myself to be 'totally awesome' and complete a superhuman feat.

Physically this change is significant, but the real strength I have found from this comes in my brain: the difference in how confident and alive I feel after a 30-minute walk is unbelievable, even though it is a slow walk on the flat! A lovely lady once told me a walk is good for the soul, and I admit that now I agree with her: after my gentle stroll I feel alive and brighter, I find myself smiling, and I think my brain and physical symptoms improve. A 30-minute walk is not inspiring, and it won't get you a Hollywood movie contract, but it will lift your spirits, and those lifted spirits may lead to you doing something amazingly inspiring. It may be that you just keep walking each day, but positivity doesn't start from sitting staring at Jeremy Kyle or Loose Women. **It begins with caring about yourself and giving your body and mind something beautiful.**

Find something that you can do to exercise the body and free the mind. It could be walking, yoga, cycling, swimming, hill walking, going to the gym or something like tai chi. Whatever your choice is, just do it, prioritise it. You may be questioning something

I wrote earlier about putting my family first and wondering how this fits with the 'prioritise your exercise' statement. Well, for a while, I didn't commit to any sort of movement every day and found myself tired, grumpy and fed up because I couldn't reach my goal of running. This wasn't my best moment, and it wasn't the most delightful experience for my family to see me sulking around.

Remember the car analogy, to treat ourselves like we do our cars: we rely on the car, and we need them increasingly in our everyday lives. So we look after them as well as we can: we use good fuel, we service them regularly, we get insurance for them and when they have had a quiet time we give them a run out otherwise the battery goes flat. This is how we should look after our bodies. We need good fuel in the form of a varied and tasty diet (note, fried food really doesn't taste as good as you think it does) and we need to get ourselves checked over by expert doctors. Life and disability insurance can help in rough times and finally, if we keep moving things we don't get rusted up.

Just think, do you care about the health of your car more than you do your own health?

I cannot prioritise my family and maintain that normality and security unless I am in the best working order possible. Hence, to ensure my family get the best from me, I must be in the best shape I can be; it is as simple as that.

**Inspiring for me is to keep positive and keep active every single day. It is not sexy or exciting, but it works. Use your Invictus Spirit and keep fighting.**

**UK cycling team**

Dave Brailsford, the performance coach of team Sky and UK cycling, had a theory: small incremental changes add up to significant 'marginal gains' in performance. I believe this is not just the way to win a three-week cycle race but also the way to live with and overcome chronic illnesses.

Brailsford is credited with championing a philosophy of 'marginal gains' at British Cycling:[23]

"The whole principle came from the idea that if you broke down everything you could think of that goes into riding a bike, and then improved it by 1%, you will get a significant increase when you put them all together" Dave Brailsford (2012)

For cycling, this might be having the same pillow and bedding every night throughout a tour, or having the same chef prepare food each night, or something as simple as ensuring your hygiene is as pristine as possible. All these small, almost insignificant aspects lead to minor improvements. Overall the small improvements can give you a substantial benefit in everyday life.

I believe this approach helps in chronic illness (I cannot afford a personal chef, although I would love one. Just imagine the variety of food, no longer just cheese sandwiches!). Little changes to how we live and mentally approach our fortunes can have substantial improvements in how we feel. Focus on the process, not the outcome: do little things today to make me feel better, and each day, the effect will accumulate. Think about it this way, if you start doing a daily walk, starting from nothing, build a plan in a 'marginal gains' way:

| Week | Walk time | How many days | Total Minutes week |
|------|-----------|---------------|--------------------|
| 1 | 5 | 4 | 20 |
| 2 | 10 | 4 | 40 |
| 3 | 15 | 4 | 60 |
| 4 | 20 | 4 | 80 |
| 5 | 20 | 5 | 100 |
| 6 | 30 | 5 | 150 |

---

[23] http://www.bbc.co.uk/sport/olympics/19174302

NOTE: Only do it if you are able; check with a healthcare professional.

By slowly increasing the daily time and then the frequency you could reach 30 minutes for five days in six weeks, and you will not notice vast differences in effort between the weeks. If you are starting from a fitter starting point, you can reach higher levels.

More simply, if you reach for an apple instead of a packet of crisps each day for a week you could save about 600 calories just by making that simple change, the idea is to make minor adjustments but keep making them.

I know we can all do some small things to make us feel more positive, whether that is just turning off the depressing daytime TV and getting outside for 20 minutes or reading a good book, instead of a rubbish magazine. It can make an enormous difference.

## Learning to trust yourself

Having confidence in yourself can be hard. It can be hard to believe in yourself when nobody else can see the symptoms; when doctors cannot find any physical explanation for your feelings, when friends tell you to pull yourself together or that you look great. It is hard to cope.

Over time, you need to learn to trust yourself. It has taken me a few years to be able to trust my own senses about when something isn't right. If I am truthful, it is a mix now of understanding my condition, understanding the normal situation and following my intuition that something is not right. I really struggled at the start and found it particularly difficult to explain my symptoms to the GP, as most were small things which, when added up, created a significant issue. Looking at the symptoms individually made me sound like a hypochondriac (which I have always tried very hard not to be). I remember saying at one point, 'I just don't feel right, but cannot explain how'. I pity the poor GP who had to deal with a comment like that; I knew it sounded stupid but did not know what else to say to him.

I can now spot worrying symptoms, and I am better able to judge when to get help and when to sleep on it and see what happens over 24 hours. I have activities at home which help to check my health: brushing my daughter's hair or walking up a flight of stairs; not difficult tasks, but they show if I am running at normal levels. However, that statement of 'I just don't feel right' still makes regular appearances at home and at the doctors, only now both my husband and the GP know this is not a good thing for me to say and they sit up and take notice.

This reaction has come about because I have (mostly) been sincere throughout and tried to not overplay the symptoms. I have kept regular (but not too frequent) contact with my GP, so he also trusts my reaction to symptoms. Again, this is about taking control of your situation as you would any other part of your life, and then using the experts for additional support.

Back to the idea of you as a car: you know how the car sounds when it is working well, and also you can spot when things are starting to break down. Whether that is squeaking brake pads or low oil, you understand a little and can detect the warning signs. You then take the car to an expert for the solution. This does not make you a car mechanic, it just means you know enough to be able to contact an expert when this is needed. It is the same with your body: you need to be able to spot your own warning signs, as nobody in the world can spot these as easily as you can. You must become knowledgeable about your condition and what is normal for you. Nobody else can tell you that your body isn't entirely running at peak performance.

I am not suggesting you become a clinical expert, I merely recommend reading the symptoms for your condition and the side effects of your treatment, and then to trust your intuition. Listen to yourself and learn to trust your feelings. When you get this right, it will give you confidence when discussing your condition with experts: it will allow you to present your feelings in a calm, factual manner, which should lead to an honest discussion about the situation and possible next steps. **It is your body, and it is your right to be involved in the decisions and options going forward, but you cannot do this if you don't understand yourself and your symptoms. I am not suggesting that you make the decisions, but that you participate fully in the discussions around your treatment.**

I hope this sounds logical, but I know that at the start, it is hard to find the confidence to trust your instincts. Unfortunately, I do not have any magic answers for this but can explain how I switched this around. As I described earlier, at the start of my journey, I really did feel that nobody believed me; in fact, to start with I don't think I believed that something was wrong. I brushed it all aside thinking that I just wasn't trying hard enough, or I was just very lazy. Part of this doubt came from the lack of clearly defined symptoms. It is easy to be confident of what is wrong when you are screaming in pain from a broken leg, but it is not so easy to explain that you had a little blood in your nose and your fingers keep shaking, and you have cold sweats and constantly waking in the night with cramp. You can convince yourself that lots of people have these symptoms and many people do, but not generally on the same day and for a prolonged period.

Vague symptoms can make you sound like a wimp trying to make a big deal out of something small, which can sound like you are a hypochondriac pulling lots of little things out of the hat, just to make it all seem worse. However, these little things can cluster into a dangerous issue, and you need to describe them all at a doctor's visit, as this will help them piece the jigsaw together. If there are lots of little things, get a pad of paper a week before your appointment and write them down as they happen (only once for each symptom, don't want to take in an essay of repeating symptoms), so that when you see the doctor, you can go through the list. If you are not comfortable listing things that you think may be silly and not related, start out with a rehearsed sentence. I always start with:

> I've listed some of the symptoms I have noticed, I am not sure if they are connected, but I would prefer to just read them to you, and then you can review all the symptoms together, and you can judge if they are connected.

This way, you are not claiming that all the items on the list are severe, or that you think that they are all part of the illness. But, if you have a good doctor, they should be able to pick up on any related to your condition. A good opening sentence that you are happy saying will help you to get all those little niggles out in the open in one go, with no need to overstate the significance of them. Be as truthful as you can be in the situation.

At the start, when I felt nobody was listening, I found myself very stressed out and exasperated with everybody and everything. This is not a healthy state of mind and probably added to my troubles. I was desperate for somebody, anybody, to confirm that my symptoms were real. This didn't happen immediately, and the lack of acknowledgement that what I was facing was real and could be treated, left me feeling very disillusioned and lonely. I found myself over-exaggerating in consultations as I thought my random symptoms were not causing the reaction I needed, so I made them seem more significant. What I probably did was make myself look over-the-top and irrational. I cried in consultations and couldn't understand how the doctors could not see how dreadful I felt; the frustration was agonising. Having the right person to listen to you is critical. A clinician must understand your illness in its totality, and for some chronic illnesses, this is a complicated process if it is a **systemic illness**, that is one that affects many parts of the body. Another word for us to learn!

Once I had referred myself to the specialist team, I went through my random list of symptoms in the first consultation and looked the consultant in the eye. I sat terrified, desperate for him to confirm I wasn't going crazy but half expecting him to react like the other doctors. It felt like hours as he looked through his notes and thought. Those few minutes of him re-reading and thinking where awful. I'm sure I forgot to breathe; the anticipation was excruciating.

When eventually he looked up from his notes and suggested I get formally transferred to him and that he believed my illness was still active, I nearly jumped up and kissed him. I did, however, manage to control myself and sit still and stay polite. The control lasted until I got into the car, and then the tears poured down my face for what seemed like hours; I just sat there crying and shaking.

The relief that somebody believed me was indescribable and signified a critical change in my life. Since that day, I have never felt the need to over-exaggerate my symptoms or look ill in a doctor's appointment again. I go in there with my usual makeup on (ladies, you know there are times when you don't put on the full war paint when visiting a doctor in case you are judged 'not to look ill'). I take my list of ALL the weird symptoms that I have faced, and I have a sensible grown-up conversation about MY condition.

It is a huge relief when somebody finally believes you, this allows you to get your confidence back. Sometimes, to get this far, you need the courage to do some research to find the right expert, or you need the determination to switch GPs and find one that you can work with effectively. I have been lucky in that respect. I had a GP that I could work with from day one, but if you do not have this crucial support move doctors NOW.

Whatever the illness, whatever part of you is affected, and whatever the future holds, you need one medical practitioner to be entirely on your side, and I would suggest that person should be your GP.  If they are not 100% on your side, you need to change.  Your journey with a chronic illness is tough, and there are many ups and downs, and probably more sidestepping than you can imagine, so it is essential to be able to go and chat to somebody who understands some of what you are going through but is not involved in your everyday life.

I hope you find the confidence and belief in yourself quickly, but if you struggle, please don't be hard on yourself.  It just takes a little time, because sometimes it's just a little bit more complicated than I have written.  I still have days when I am not sure if I need to react and contact somebody or just rest, but now I rarely panic about it because usually, these are the days when things are borderline 'just rest/contact doctor'.  On these days, I have learnt to go to sleep and reassess how I feel in 24 hours.  It usually then becomes apparent what I need to do.  Advice is always helpful.  I often ask my husband if he thinks I am worse than the week before because I try to look on the positive side and make out that I am better than I really am.

**It is imperative to learn to trust your intuition and not to be too hard on yourself if you get things wrong or make the wrong choices.  It is a learning process and, there is always more to learn.  I am still guilty of doing too much when I start to feel a bit better.  I feel all excited, start planning lots of things, racing to be back to normal, and then 48 hours later I am reminded in an obvious way that life has changed and I will not be back to my old self anytime soon, if ever.**

My GP, who had been with me from the beginning recently retired.  It was an enormous shock (as I didn't think he was that old) and I felt really lost again.  Currently I have been assigned to two new GPs who job share, and I am building up my trust and relationship with them.  However, if the relationship does not become strong within a year, I will be requesting a change, as I know the importance of a good GP supporting you through the crap times and I don't want to have a doctor that I cannot trust with my life.

**Find somebody to rant to.**

The previous section talked about learning to trust yourself, and this is important, but you also need somebody who you can happily share all your emotions with. If you cannot share your feelings with somebody, it will be challenging to understand them. I'm great at holding in my emotions, this is not always a good plan. I have great conversations with myself about the future. The problem with these conversations in my head is that there isn't any 'sanity check' on the ideas; my brain metaphorically runs away with itself.

Now a good daydream is excellent, but when you start to believe these extremes, it becomes slightly more worrying. My dreams about my future plans vary wildly from day to day. One day I will want to get a nanny in and go full on back to work, rising to the top of the company. The next day (when I have been over-excited the day before) I cannot cope with it all and want to give up and be self-employed, controlling the days I work. Neither day is my real dream, but they feel incredibly real at the time, and I am determined they are what I want on that day.

When your brain is affected by the treatment, the concern over the future the illness will leave you with, or by generally feeling terrible, it is challenging to make the right choice and be sure about your decisions. If you can hold off on major decisions, please do postpone until you can make a rational choice, often this will only be a couple of days later.

The danger comes when we cannot notice these swings or extremes. I know I have these swings, and I try and make sure that I don't react to any 'new ideas' for at least 24 hours, to try and ensure it isn't just my brain making plans I will never be able to keep.

I am getting better at understanding these. Although I have been known to order books from Amazon for a new plan, and by the time I have got them through the letterbox, the idea seems ridiculous. I find the best test is to tell somebody what I have been plotting. If I can finish the words without realising that it sounds silly, then my trusted 'sounding board' will soon let me know what they think. I have some excellent sounding boards, each with their own specific skills and place in my life, and I couldn't be without them. Talking about and physically sharing my thoughts helps me process them and brings them into reality, which also helps to put some practical constraints on them. When you are physically hindered, it can be very easy to feel isolated and lonely, and it can be hard for others to understand that the illness adds a new dimension to all the other problems you may face.

Having a chronic illness, a permanently changed life, (maybe) reduced contact with friends and colleagues, and taking medication that can interfere with your emotional state, all mean that it is imperative that you have a trusted person you can talk to about anything. The conversations don't have to be heavy; it could be just that you giggle about something silly, or it might be that they have had similar experiences and so can offer practical advice as well as excellent listening skills. Just do not lock yourself away and hold everything inside.

Remember the comments from an earlier chapter: friendships need to be a two-way partnership, at least over the longer term, so make sure the conversations are not only about your illness or concerns. It would take an exceptional friend to listen just to your negatives and never to be able to share their comments. You are not the only person with problems, and it will do you lots of good to listen to other people's issues as well as your own. Just remember it isn't a competition over who has the worst life/symptom/partner... even if you feel you could win the competition hands down.

**One of my biggest rants is the fact that I am sooooooo bored of being ill; this is a recurring subject for me. It is difficult for people to understand how draining it can be to wake up every day and feel ill for many years. I find the whole thing boring now, but this is life, and I don't expect it to change.**

So, I have a rant about it, it usually only lasts a few minutes over coffee, and then I move on to other things. The rant gets rid of the frustration. I cannot really change this frustration, so voicing it and leaving it behind works for me. Maybe you will find a different way to deal with this frustration.

I find the rants stop the emotions building up too much. There will always be times when everything gets too much, and I go off in a corner and cry, but those moments are reducing, and I'm happy with the ratio of:

Good days: Rant days: Down days

I believe we must accept a mix of the three types of days, but if the ratio moves too far to the right, you may want to think about getting extra help to move the ratio back to the left and restore your balance.

**Down days are part of a chronic illness; even the most positive of us will have days where we feel rubbish about everything (people WITHOUT a chronic illness also have these, remember not everything can be blamed on the illness). It is how we pick ourselves up and deal with the bad days that shows how we are coping with the changes. Having a few down days does not make you depressed; having a chronic illness does not make you depressed, and having a rant doesn't make you depressed.**

However, if we have a change in life or live with an illness, we can be prone to depression, stress or anxiety. That is fine, and if you feel you have more down days than you think you should, again you should be proactive and go and talk to your GP. Do not try and fight it on your own, there are amazing support tools out there to help us.

The world looks at depression very differently than it did ten years ago, and we seem to understand it a lot more. There is a lot of support out there, but you must tell somebody how you feel before anybody knows that you need assistance. It is not easy to ask for help, but if you are starting to feel low, you must go and seek help to get some support. Think about your current ratio of Good: Rant: Down days; is it moving to the right of the equation?. There is a website from the NHS that is great for helping you to assess your true feelings. I am not saying that this is a diagnosis, but it will help you to realise if it is time to talk to somebody:

http://www.nhs.uk/Conditions/stress-anxiety-depression/Pages/low-mood-and-depression.aspx

Six years into my illness and I felt the need for emotional support, as I was struggling with the body had I been left with after the illness and the treatment. My GP managed to get me somebody to talk too within a few weeks, so different from the 18month wait I was told about at the beginning of my journey with this illness. They helped me realise that it is not unusual to have the feelings I have, and also gave me simple, practical ways to try and move forward. I knew this time that I didn't want anti-depressant tablets, I needed breathing space and time to talk and process what I am left with.

If you struggle, please find help, it can be a fantastic comfort, I found that just describing the start of my illness in the conversation started me crying again, which surprised me as I thought I had dealt with the early days. Obviously, I still had raw emotions from the whole journey.

Chronic illness leaves us all fed up sometimes, and it makes it difficult to deal with everything that is thrown at us. So if you feel down and a good rant isn't helping, don't be hard on yourself. You are not the only one in this situation, and you are not the only one feeling fed up. So don't beat yourself up, but calmly take a step back and have a look at things from a different angle; how can you help yourself? If you can find a way to help yourself, even just a little, then you are taking control back and will feel a small amount of positivity, and hopefully, that will grow.

But remember, if you are feeling low go and talk to your doctor; don't sit there and let it take over you. There is no shame in admitting you are struggling a little or a lot, we all do. Some of us struggle more than others and need additional support. Remember you would instantly go to get help if you broke your leg, so why not when your head is not working smoothly.

**Patient associations**

I am a member of a patient association, and it has been a great support and source of knowledge for me. I am very grateful for everything it has done over the years. It is run by some incredibly knowledgeable and passionate people, who are truly amazing (and they are all volunteers, which is even more amazing). Do not misunderstand anything I am about to write. I am not against patient associations; they are invaluable in giving patients real-world knowledge and experience of a particular illness. They help you connect with others in the same situation and maybe facilitate a meeting for a cup of coffee if that is what you want. Join the Facebook page and learn and share, but do not feel pressure to be actively posting or contributing.

Patient associations also wield power with governments, medical companies and doctors; they can help to support you if you feel you are not getting the treatment you need, and they can offer advice regarding money issues, government benefits and other problems you may face. So, join one and use the information and support they can provide you on your journey. But, also be a little cautious. Most people working with patient associations are well trained and knowledgeable, and their main aim is to help you cope with your illness.

However, some members may not be so confident. You can see this clearly on some Facebook or other social media sites, where feedback amongst patients can get a little bitchy if you don't all agree, or patients start to 'diagnose' other patients online without all the facts. We have all heard it: 'My mum's neighbour has that, and she swears that, if she sits with feet up for 48 hours, it all goes away', or 'You should try the Paleo diet, it can cure you within days'. I don't know if either of these things works, I haven't researched them or asked my doctor, but I do know that I have never heard any of my doctors recommend the Paleo diet!

The danger starts when you are not sure what is helpful advice and support, and what is from somebody who may quite enjoy telling you stories that have no evidence. It can be tempting to let your life become consumed entirely by being ill. People may be well-meaning and may be genuinely trying to help you, but they do not know your individual medical history and they are often not medically trained, though they may imply they are experts. When we are desperate for answers, we will take any advice given to us from a kind person. You need to stay sensible if something sounds like it will cure you, but your doctors have not mentioned it, then question what evidence is available. It is not a conspiracy by the Pharmaceutical companies, but it is probably because there is no evidence to show that it makes any difference. Clinical trials have been run on nutrition supplements and alternative medicines (contrary to what some say in the press), so if there is any benefit to be achieved for your illness, your doctor will be aware of it. Therefore you should discuss what you have heard or been told with them. No doctor is trying to keep you ill to sell pharmaceutical products.

**Above all else, do not change or stop your treatment on the advice of other patients. They do not know your personal history and therefore are not able to offer completely safe advice.**

For me, one of the hardest things about chronic illness is trying to stay positive. Some days I fail miserably at this one task, and often on those days, I feel I need to rant. An effortless way to rant is to post something on social media. I have done this in the past, just a few sentences about how fed up I am and how I wish there were an answer; I think this is normal. I had never thought about how this would affect others in the social media group. Selfishly I just thought I would get some support or sympathy in return for my 'honest' post. The problem is that this wasn't really an 'honest' post; well, it *was* honest for the 30 minutes before and after I posted it.

But in reality, after I posted the comment and then had a cup of coffee and re-read the comments, I sort of started to pull myself back together and no longer felt the same way. Great, I solved MY misery. Looking back now, I wonder what effect this had on others in the group; did it cause them to despair or lose their positivity for the day? I don't know, but I am sure it didn't have a positive effect on those who read my words.

I tend to post things online when either life seems bad, or I have just had some devastating news, or on days when I am brimming with positivity. These are all the extremes of my emotions that are not representative of my on-going life with a chronic illness. These are the moments when things seem impossible, so I need to share them to help me cope with them. The problem is that if we only ever post the extremes of emotions, then that is all people will see. They don't observe the days when I am giggling with my children or trying to stay resilient in a work meeting. I don't share any of these every day almost 'mundane' experiences with a social media group. I am pretty certain that I am not the only one who shares only the worst or best of my experiences.

So if you are new to illness and are reading the posts, you may start to think your world has collapsed and that this is going to be the most awful illness ever seen. But your world won't cave in; you need to remember you are reading about everybody's 'worst days'. You need to try and keep some perspective on the posts and remember that, though these may be happening to 100 different people, you may only have to face one of the dreadful things posted, which may be easy to deal with in its isolation. Please don't start obsessing that all the issues discussed will affect you.

My husband always says that I am a competitive mum. This comes from a question I ask at each parents evening: 'Is she where she should be in comparison to others?' I don't believe this is competitive. In business, we call it 'benchmarking': comparing yourself to others to analyse how well you are doing. I believe we all do this in our lives and nowhere is this more apparent than on social media; we check-in and post pictures showing how amazing our life is at that moment in time. Well, I notice that on some social media health sites, it can become a sort of competition of who has the worst story. It is a little similar to new mums who sit in a coffee shop and discuss the birth; it nearly always becomes a discussion around who had the most horrendous birth. It is natural, and I am sure some very clever people can explain the theory behind this, but it gives us a small insight into what can happen on social media. We are not in competition; we need to support each other with honesty and try not to 'out symptom' each other in our responses. I have seen genuine requests for advice met with the line, 'but my symptoms are severe.' The person was asking for advice on a different issue to the answer the person gave. I suspect the responder needed to rant for themselves and indeed wrote the comment to rant rather than support the person with the original question.

One more note on online forums: I have seen a lot of comments about the use of 'natural therapies', where people often quote that natural cannot do you any harm. Be a little careful; remember nettles are natural, but you don't want to rub them on your skin, Hemlock grows naturally but is highly poisonous. **Natural does not equal Safe. As with medication, do your research and talk to medical professionals; make sure you check out the qualification of any alternative therapist you turn to. If they tell you to stop your prescription medicine, walk away and, if you have the strength, report them to the medicines' authorities. Remember you are responsible for making sure you get the best treatment, so be sure to research thoroughly any options you consider taking.**

Patient associations are an integral part of our journey; they are truly amazing organisations that can fight for our best interests and offer us the kind of support that a clinician cannot, because they understand the impact on our life and not just the medical implications. They can, if you choose, become a significant part of our life, or we can sit quietly on the edge, observing others interact. It is our choice. However, you utilise the benefits, find a way that is right for you. But **don't** change any medication or treatment because of any advice you get without discussing with your doctor; don't get 'symptom competitiveness', but try to share an accurate reflection of your battle so that others realise that life is not just the extremes of emotions. And don't judge how others react and cope with their journeys, it is all individual.

## Everybody has their own battles

Six years of waking up each day feeling awful, some days terrible others a little better; it is easy to think this is a never-ending battle. Your life can become consumed by being ill or consumed by ways of trying to feel better and stay positive. At times, I admit, I have simply forgotten the rest of the world: if I managed to get the kids to school and get back home without having to discuss my illness with… this seemed like a roaring success.

Until …

You realise that you have become so self-obsessed with your fight and symptoms, that you are missing important events in your friends' lives. You forget that friends need you as much as you need them. My most shocking realisation was when a friend mentioned flippantly how poorly her father had become; I was genuinely shocked; I didn't even know he was ill. I had been so preoccupied with my chemo treatment and how awful that had been making me feel, that I had retreated away from friends and, as a result, I wasn't there when I was needed. I felt guilty and apologised, and of course, my friend said I had nothing to apologise for. But I disagree, I could have been there for her. I had great first-hand experience of how the healthcare system worked that may have helped, or we could have just sat and cried or cursed together.

When I am ill, I tend to pull back from friends and stay at home. For example, when you go through toxic treatment, it is very easy to lock yourself away and virtually give up on your social life. This may be a great short-term strategy to help you get stronger, healthier or maybe to avoid infection, but it can leave you lonely and cut off in the longer term.

Initially, people will try and come and see you and make exceptions, but memories are short, especially if your illness is invisible, and the lives of others move on. Good friends don't run away, but their lives continue; if you lock yourself away, you will become less and less part of those lives. This isn't a planned exclusion; it is just that people move on and become part of a new social circle, and you may not be included as you are not there to join in the conversation.

There is a balance, a sensible balance between prioritising your friends and ensuring you look after yourself. Remember that while your problems are real, so are your friend's issues. They have health risks, family fall outs and their own worries, and you cannot expect them to listen only to you and your problems. I may be stating the obvious here, and if you feel I am patronising you, then I apologise; you are a better friend than I have been. However, some of you will recognise yourself in these comments and start to realise that outside of your own issues, you are not 'in the loop' with your friends anymore. I have seen online posts really laying into friends for wanting to talk about something other than the person's illness, or comments that friends don't understand how hard it is for us every day. I think it is unfair to judge friends for not understanding, as I don't think it is possible to understand the impact a chronic illness can have until you have to live with it daily. Your friends are not thoughtless, but they may not understand. The best way for them to understand is for you to talk to them and share your feelings and you listen to their opinions in return.

Get back out there today. That is the only answer: get back out and see people, talk, and make sure you listen properly to your friends; you need them, and they need you.

Once I realised that I had been backing out of lots of things, my husband and I promised each other that we would stop cancelling going out even if I felt a bit rough; we would go and see how things went. We reasoned that we could always leave early if I felt terrible. Sometimes we left early and sometimes I got some mysterious energy from a secret store and lasted most of the night.

STOP!

I can hear some shouts as you are reading this, 'Well it's ok for her to go out, I can't get out!' It wasn't ok for me to go out. I often felt awful throughout the event, and I always had payback for the energy consumed; probably 24 hours of extreme fatigue or an afternoon in bed, or even a temperature which meant I had a slight infection somewhere. If I had a few alcoholic beverages, then the payback would be greatly exaggerated, and I could be wiped out for days. I took the decision to try and return to a little of my old life and do these ordinary social events, being acutely aware that I would have to deal with the consequences over the next few days. For me this is worth it: to have a night where I feel full of fun and mischief again is a revitalising feeling.

Only you can make the decisions about how to get the balance right, knowing all your circumstances. But having some fun can really lift our mood.

Socialising doesn't have to mean drinking or nights out, two of my favourite days in the last few years have been visits to a spa, once with my mother-in-law and the other with old friends from school. Nice relaxing days with lots of pampering and no exertion or alcohol necessary (although my friends drank enough to cover my rations). Spa breaks are no longer just for women: I went to a place called Hoar Cross Hall, and in the evening, there was about a 60:40 Women: Men. So go and be pampered; male or female, you deserve a rest. If you are there all day, you all have plenty of time to share your issues, so there is no rush to get your issues in first.

What a great way to look after yourself and really get a connection back with your friends, sharing problems from both sides.

Another problem I have found with having an illness is that my memory doesn't seem to work as efficiently as it used too. Or maybe it is having two children, or just that I am getting older. Who knows? See, I told you it is dangerous to always blame issues on the illness; it could be just that I am getting older. Initially, I found myself missing birthdays or school shows. Life just became a little harder to manage and plan, so again, I had to change how I organised myself (and the family).

I used the paper calendar more, I set reminders on my phone and in my work calendar, and I just wrote things down physically. I sent birthday presents direct to the person and got the company to wrap them. This saved me having to physically wrap and travel to the post office (I know this sounds quite impersonal, but I think it is better that friends get a present rather than I spend weeks building up the energy to make it to the post office).

Good friends understand this, and those that don't, well, you shouldn't be sending presents to them anyway ;-). I learnt that children over the age of four years LOVE to receive vouchers for Argos or Claire's accessories, and I become a regular on Amazon and Click-and-Collect services. The thought of a day out shopping made me feel sick. It is all about smart shopping now: buying in advance so I have time to find the energy to wrap or sending directly with wrapping done for me, still thoughtful but just a little smarter.

Social interaction is critical in making you feel at your best. Often, I find when I go out with my pretend smile on my face, it turns quite quickly into a real smile, and this is accompanied by giggles and my old cheekiness. This is always a good recipe for making me feel better inside. Spending time with friends will get you back involved, and you can all take it in turns to be the shoulder to cry on. Isolation can intensify your feelings and make them seem bigger: the longer you stay isolated, the greater the feelings appear, so share them. The old saying of 'a problem shared is a problem halved' is correct.

Keep talking and listening, and you will probably start to quite enjoy being back out in the real world; I know I have. Always allow yourself time to rest before or after the events. When I had a party for my 40th birthday, we had friends travelling for hours to get there. Usually, I would have let them stay at our house, and then we could have carried on after the official party had finished. On this occasion, I was awaiting treatment, and we weren't even sure I would make the party. So we were selfish: we didn't let anybody stay with us, and I slept for a long time on the day of the party so that I could 'sparkle' in the evening. A bit of forward planning and selfishness allowed me to celebrate in style, and none of my friends was in the slightest bit offended.

## Fragility

Fragility is a delightful word that provides a perfect description for living with a chronic illness. The Oxford English Dictionary describes fragility as:

*(Of a person) not strong or sturdy; delicate and vulnerable*

I spend a significant number of my days feeling delicate and vulnerable. I do not find it a comfortable state of mind, but one that I face and try to live with. The illness has left me physically and mentally delicate and vulnerable. I remain very stubborn, ambitious and driven, so to be left feeling these fragile emotions make me feel threatened, angry, scared and very, very frustrated. This feeling is hard to describe to friends and family, as their reaction is to try and make you feel better about the changes. It is difficult for others to understand that because of this fragility, you spend a significant amount of time pretending to be ok: the smile comes out, and you avoid showing the weakness you feel daily. The consequence of 'pretending for a day' is exhaustion, as it takes a lot of physical and emotional energy to keep up the façade; you hide away on bad days and only show the physical smile that is faked. I avoid explaining these feelings to friends as it sounds like you are trying to 'trick' them with pretence, but it is not about tricking anybody else. It is about trying to fool yourself into believing you are strong, and fighting and winning when, in reality, it is hard to think this when facing another relapse or another awkwardly embarrassing medical examination.

Another reason for not telling people how fragile I feel is because, once they know, it is virtually impossible to hide the fragility from them going forward. I have been reluctant to reveal my strategy of hiding with all my friends because the plan will not work as well in the future. Some of you will be reading this and shouting that I should share it with all my friends, and maybe you are right. I have a couple of friends who are fully aware of my fragility and who also respect my right to still hide it without them pointing it out to everybody. However, remember this book is not about giving you a plan; it is about sharing my lessons learned and decisions made so you can make a more informed decision about how best to cope in similar situations. My thought is that if I can act as healthy as possible then maybe, just maybe, I will have a level of normality, no matter how fragile I feel on that day.

Strangely, nothing makes me feel more vulnerable than the phrase:

*But you look so well*

I really struggle when people say this to me, and yes, I am aware that they are saying it with kind thoughts and genuinely positively mean this statement. Let me try to explain how it makes me feel. I try to look healthy and well; some days, I succeed, and some days, I look dreadful. I can deal with that. I don't think I am a vain person, but the physical changes of weight gain, swollen face and a generally knackered look do have a negative effect on my mood. So, in a way when somebody says 'but you look so well,' I know I should be flattered, I know they are nice. But it always feels a little like they have missed the end of the sentence off, and in my mind the end of the sentence is one of these …

> … are you sure you are not better?
>
> … I'm not sure what you keep moaning about
>
> … that maybe it is in your head
>
> … you can't really be that ill if you can have your nails and hair done
>
> … come on pull yourself together and stop milking it

I know that my friends don't mean anything like this, but I'm sure some acquaintances really do think these things as they make the flippant comment. That is up to them; I cannot change what they believe, and I know I shouldn't care about their impression of me. However, these comments make me feel more vulnerable.

I want to stand in the schoolyard and shout:

## I AM ALLOWED TO LOOK WELL. IT DOES NOT MEAN I AM CURED OR RUNNING A MARATHON OR MAKING IT ALL UP. I JUST LOOK OK TODAY!

Obviously, I don't shout this as I am not a rude person (and my children would be so embarrassed if I did), but some days it really does cross my mind. It is very tempting to explain that often how I look on the outside does not correlate with how I feel on the inside. Some days they are linked and others they are the polar opposite; I often hide how dreadful I feel with make-up. So please don't judge the severity or activity of my illness by whether I look well groomed or not on that day.

Fragile is a delicate word that describes perfectly how my chronic illness makes me feel. I wish it didn't, but that is how this awful illness leaves me: fragile, vulnerable and delicate.

**But I'm not destroyed, I still put up a feeble fight, striving for normality and happy, positive life. That is why I choose to bury my fragility under my smile; to ensure I face each day with a willingness and enthusiasm to fight and keep my Invictus spirit; to battle every day, and just 'keep going' in the life I have at this moment.**

Simple things can cause huge upheaval. On one hospital visit for a routine appointment, I ended up leaving the building six and a half hours later. Maybe it is some great marketing scam by the NHS to sell the food in the hospital and boost funds, but I don't think they are sophisticated enough to plan that.

I entered the hospital to get the results from my latest heart scan, which were stable in comparison with last year's results. After a mess up with the appointment bookings, my 11am appointment became a 12 appointment. Then the consultant was running 90 minutes late as some idiot had booked all the appointments in for the morning. The consultant and nurse were apologetic, and it is hard to get annoyed at somebody who had nothing to do with the planning. But it still meant that my whole day involved waiting around.

When I finally saw the consultant, she was concerned as I had a burst a blood vessel in my eye. Because of my condition, this could have been something serious, so I was added to another clinic list. Therefore, after I had my blood samples taken, I then sat for over an hour to wait to get my simple bloodshot eye checked out. It turned out to be a normal bloodshot eye, which healed by itself within a few days.

I got home exhausted, fed up and a day behind on work. The time it takes to see doctors, visit clinics, and have all the necessary tests can be underestimated and not fully understood by employers. I brought work to do with me, but it isn't possible to get much done sitting on a small plastic chair in a drafty corridor that doubles up as a waiting room.

**Having a chronic illness sometimes feels like a full-time job**: getting medicines, measuring them out for the week, visiting GPs, visiting clinics, having tests, going for the regular blood tests, remembering flu jabs and precautionary treatments…all leave you feeling very fragile. But all the monitoring and caution is necessary because as much as I hate to admit it, I am vulnerable and dull things like a cold can take many weeks to recover from or leave me in a hospital for weeks and so Doctors always double check things. Unfortunately.

## Invisible illness

Many chronic illnesses are invisible, which adds an extra complication to the journey.

Simply, this means that you look normal, not ill, like nothing serious is happening; which isn't the reality. There are advantages and disadvantages to the illness being invisible: it means that you can carry on and hide it from friends and strangers, and it can be easier to shelter your family from reality. If people don't see the illness, it can also mean that you don't have to continually discuss it and you can 'introduce' it only to those people that you want to be aware of your suffering. You can go out and eat with friends and nobody will know; you will not get any stares from people wondering what is wrong, as there is be no obvious evidence of your troubles. People may be able to see the side effects of some treatment, such as weight gain or loss, but they cannot see your physical or mental illness inside. But the effects are always there for you, and that is very hard to deal with constantly.

These are some of the positive aspects of invisible illnesses, but invisibility is a double-edged sword.

One disadvantage is that people do not know you are ill unless you tell them; I'm not very good at talking about my personal condition. I like to deflect the conversations back to being about the other person, so the initial conversation with someone about being ill is still the hardest conversation for me. I have a few 'stock' sentences that I use when starting the discussion, but it is still difficult to tell people about my struggles.

Having young children that are invited to lots of parties meant that I started to become quite open with the other parents because I rarely made it to the parties, or the school social events and I didn't want people to think that I was rude. I needed to show that there was a physical reason for my absence (again praise must be given to my husband for going to so many little girls' birthday parties, which I know he didn't always enjoy). I found myself sharing things on Facebook as it was easier for me to write how I felt and include links to facts about my rare illness. I hope people didn't find these updates depressing but understood that I found this a 'less intimate' way of sharing the details; also it helps friends who I don't regularly see to know where I am with everything.

After the initial diagnosis, when people are so keen to help you and offer support, people cannot see the illness, and you continue as normally as you can, so people can simply forget you are ill. Some assume that all is cured, others are busy enjoying their life and forget about your 'hiccup', and some just think all must be ok because you look normal. The dilemma comes from trying to decide whether you remind people that you are living with an illness for life or just let it be forgotten.

The decision depends on the illness, the severity of the symptoms, you as a person and how open you want to be about your battle; and, of course, how important the friendship is to you. I don't think this is an easy decision and it may depend on how you feel in the split second that somebody says, 'how are you?'. I admit that I find it surprising that sometimes emotions come out stronger than I expect, and often this happens with the least likely of people - people I may not initially know very well. However, once my emotions have surfaced, and the conversation becomes a sincere one, they do seem to become good friends.

We don't like to imagine that people suffer daily battles and if we do not see the suffering or the impact of the battles, we tend to put the knowledge to the back of our brains and ignore the fact that the person faces a long-term illness. I try not to judge those who do this, I think I am guilty of this to some extent with my friends.

There are many things that you can control: who do you tell, how do you tell them, and should you keep reminding them or discussing your challenges, or just let the memory drift away.

The next challenge with invisible illnesses is that some people just do not believe you are ill. This is extremely hard; I hope it comes from people not understanding the challenges, rather than malicious thoughts. The people who do not believe you may be friends or family, which is hard enough, but it becomes more upsetting when you are trying to convince doctors and employers that even though you look fine, you feel terrible. Patient associations can help in this situation; many have material that you can use to explain your hidden symptoms. Use them, in fact, use every resource you can find. YouTube has short video clips of anything you want to find, so share the (good) links and let somebody else explain the feelings and symptoms you have. It will help show that you are not alone; often, these videos are very cleverly written and really do help to improve understanding. Also, it will help you feel like you aren't the one moaning or after sympathy.

When people don't believe you, it becomes very tempting to exaggerate your symptoms and the impact they have on your everyday life. I have done this, as it felt like the only way I would be believed. Unfortunately, this over-exaggeration does not convince experienced doctors. **Exaggerating your symptoms is not a good plan;** exaggeration can very quickly become like the 'pretend smile' turning into a 'real smile'.

If you overplay your symptoms to make people believe you, eventually you may find yourself believing these new more substantial symptoms yourself. It is tempting, and I have done it occasionally, but in the long term, it is not a healthy plan. It is much better to do a little research and find an expert in your field and visit them. Remember, it is vital that you take control of the situation, and don't let things control you, so that believe the only way forward is to over-emphasise your symptoms.

Invisible illnesses have positives and negatives compared to illnesses that are obvious to those around you. The trick is to use the positives to your advantage and learn how to live with the negatives, remembering that it really does not matter what those people outside of your close family really think. It is difficult, but any doubters can just go and annoy somebody else; you know your issues are real.

# Rare Diseases

All chronic illnesses are scary, emotional and challenging. However when you then add the complication of being 'rare', things can get even more confusing.

- A rare illness is defined by the European Union as one that affects less than five in 10,000 of the general population;
- There are between 6,000 and 8,000 known rare illnesses;
- Around five new rare illnesses are described in medical literature each week;
- One in 17 people, or 7% of the population, will be affected by a rare illness at some point in their lives;
- This equates to approximately 3.5 million people in the UK and 30 million people across Europe;
- In the UK, a single rare illness may affect up to about 30,000 people. The vast majority of rare illnesses will affect far fewer than this – some will affect only a handful or even a single person in the whole of the UK;
- 80% of rare illnesses have a genetic component; and
- Often rare illnesses are chronic and life-threatening.[24]

The NHS is excellent at dealing with 'common' issues. They have care pathways which outline the routes to follow for the treatment of specified problems. Although these routes can sometimes feel frustrating for the patient, you at least feel like you are being treated with confidence and with a proven process.

For patients with rare illnesses, this confidence in the treatment can be missing, and often, your GP will never have seen a person with your illness. So your GP cannot offer much advice in the way of medical options, they can still provide you with all the support you need in every other way and if they don't, start looking for another one.

Your local hospital may not have had much experience with your specific problems, and so they may not be the best place to get treated. All this adds to the fearfulness of living with an illness.

---

[24] http://www.rareillness.org.uk/about-rare-illnesses.htm

I have a rare illness and, I had to take control of my treatment: I had to do a little research and transfer myself to a hospital that was a centre of excellence. I won't say this was an unproblematic process. The analysis was easy; you can search the patient associations and see which medical advisors they use or look at any clinical papers they mention or just ask the patient association if they can tell you the centre of excellence closest to your home. The hard bit comes from believing you should request the transfer and the guilt you feel from 'betraying' your current doctors.

Having gone through the process, I must say that if you feel that your medical team do not know enough about your condition, you have every right to request to be seen by experts.

With rare illnesses, this is critical, as they are illnesses which non-specialists may not have exposure to or experience of dealing with effectively. It is similar to making a cake: the first time you make it, it will not be brilliant (no matter how good a cook you think you are). The second time it may be better, but if you make it every day, you will know if it will be right before you put it in the oven and you will also know what small changes you can make to the recipe to improve it or alter the taste to suit.

If a doctor sees one patient with a condition they are basing their decisions on what they have read, but if they talk to patients every week or every month then they are basing decisions on their real-life experience, and the expertise gained, as well as the published evidence. **You have a right to be seen by a medical team who are experienced in dealing with your specific problems. Simple as that.**

So, what do you do? You find the place you want to go, considering the distance you will need to travel and how you will get to and from appointments. I am happy to drive an hour each way, though sometimes it feels like a pain, but, when I have active illness, I am so glad I can speak to experts. It is an acceptable trade-off for getting a team supporting me that I trust and believe in. Decide what is acceptable for you, you need to take control of this and decide what is right. Your decision will depend on the illness, where you live, what kind of support you have from friends and family, and how often you will need to travel to the hospital/clinic.

Talk to your GP about the fact you are thinking of switching doctors, they can help you. I spoke with my GP, and the doctor I wanted to transfer from was well known to them, and they had mutual respect. I had to explain that I wasn't criticising the doctor, I was merely requesting to see somebody with more specialist knowledge of my illness. I tried to keep it factual rather than emotional, even though I really wanted to shout, 'he just doesn't get it!'.

By keeping it factual about knowledge rather than about the individual, you can put your argument forward in a calm, persuasive manner.

Your GP should then write to the centre of excellence, or your chosen site, requesting they meet with you. For me, this involved a long conversation with the specialist, which ended in them accepting me as a patient. The day was so emotional, and I felt I was betraying my old doctor.

I was terrified the new doctor would tell me it was all in my head. I thought maybe my illness wasn't serious enough for me to be requesting this change. So many conflicting thoughts. It was all worth it for me when the expert said they would take me on and that they were confident that the illness was still active. Pure relief flooded throughout my body.

Rare illnesses receive less publicity, less fundraising, less research and less investment from government and industry. This is a fact of life and probably correct as they affect fewer people, but there needs to be investment and research and focus on rare illnesses. Just because an illness is rare does not mean that the person dealing with it faces less impact on their lives. I don't believe that the balance is quite right at present. This is changing, and rare illnesses are seeing investment, but it will take a while to catch up for the years of neglect. Fingers crossed that as this 'catch-up' happens some significant discoveries happen.

**How about we fund more general services which are not dependent on the type of illness faced by the patients?**

Another issue with a rare illness is the knowledge about the effects of the illness on you. Your friends will not be aware of the impact, and you cannot just say, 'I've been diagnosed with xxxxx' and expect them to understand. It is not the same as something like diabetes, where people can realise straightaway the implications and treatments you will encounter.

With rare illnesses, you may have to spend time explaining the journey you face, which can be hard. I got around this by sharing links on social media. I didn't want to spend most of my days explaining everything I have to deal with. Don't get annoyed if people don't understand, just remember that before you were diagnosed, you didn't understand either.

It is not because people do not want to comprehend, rather, the information may not be there or not very easy to read. Have patience.

Recently I have given in and ordered a medical alert bracelet. I pretended for a long time that I really don't need this failsafe. Again, I have been naïve; this little bracelet (and there many choices available) will tell the emergency services my issues in an instant and may well be a true lifesaver in the same way it is for people with severe allergies. Also, it is an excuse for wearing more bracelets day-to-day to make it less noticeable! Be safe and buy one if you need one, so if you are treated, and you are unconscious, the medical practitioners will know a small but critical part of your clinical history.

One final comment about rare illnesses: it is critical that you try and understand the illness a little, as you will often face doctors who do not fully understand it. On a trip to A&E, there is nothing worse than a doctor looking at you with no understanding of your illness. You need to be an expert in your situation if only to stop any unnecessary treatment or tests from those who do not understand. If you struggle with this, go to the patient association and print off a short summary about your illness and how it is treated, write down your medications and any specifics you have faced, and keep it all with you so that you can hand it over if you need to in an emergency.

## My personal thoughts on …

### Industry

I have heard many discussions about how the medical industry should face the challenges of chronic illness, and about how they should consult with patients and patient associations.

After reading the discussions in journals about how to deal with patients, I cannot decide if I find this focus funny or frustrating. To me, there is no discussion to have: diagnosed patients are no different to the people manufacturing and selling the products or services that can help us. The only difference between the manufacturer and patient may be that our illness has shown its cards, and we have been diagnosed with an illness. I am the same person I was six years ago, but I have additional challenges, and I have also gained further insight into these challenges.

My illness has not created an entirely new person, and I have not become a clone to match everybody else with my illness. Each person with my illness faces a diverse set of personal challenges; some may be similar, but each person still is unique.

My illness does not mean that I am the same as all the other people with my illness; I still don't like driving at night, I love good full-fat macaroni cheese, I prefer to drink red wine. And I believe passionately that Jaffa cakes are the best thing ever invented. It is very simple from me to industry:

**Find a cure for me without side-effects, please.**

If this is not currently possible then work towards it, work to understand my illness in a way I cannot: study it, review past studies, review available drugs to see if they could work for me, look at the biology, chemistry, physics and any other scientific discipline you can find for my illness. Use every bit of knowledge available to search for the cure.

I think this sounds logical, and at a human level, it is; do everything within your power to find a cure. *Please*.

As a world, we do not work together to find a cure. Egos, politics, intellectual property, patents, competition, money, they all get in the way to prevent collaborative working. Scientific knowledge is not commonly shared; profits decide which work gets started, and patents, profits and politics decide if trials are continued, and whether something that could save my life is investigated through to a final manufactured product or if it stays as a promising laboratory study.

If you work in medical research, materials research or electronics, or any related subject, please think about what you are doing; think about the impact this could have on my life. What if you were diagnosed tomorrow, how would you approach things then? **This is my message to the industry: really think about what a small amount of extra urgency could contribute. Could it save one or ten lives over the next day or month? This might not sound much, but that could be 360 people a year... for the next 10 years. So please work with urgency, break down the rules and politics that stop us sharing work, and work to eradicate many of today's illnesses.**

Do it because, even if you cannot get motivated to help others, you may be the next to be diagnosed. So do it for yourself today while you are still able to work. *Please*.

**Patient-Centric?**

I have seen articles written about the industry being 'Patient Centric'. Surely, by definition, the medical industry exists to be 'patient-centric' because what else should it focus on ... surely, its purpose is to help treat and cure people with an illness?

Financiers will be jumping up and down about how there are shareholders and investors. Yes, I am aware that businesses need money, and people need to make money from investing in these hugely profitable companies. But as a global population, we should really consider the implication of this, are the companies who decide which drugs or devices to develop to the final product really focused on curing the patient, or making profits for the already wealthy investors?

If the focus is profits, then they can never be totally patient-centric, which is fine, as they are private companies and, as such, do not really have any obligations to me as a patient. Being patient-centric means putting the patient's well-being at the centre of your decisions, which is not always an easy option. It is not just holding a conference where you 'let patients tell you their stories'.

To me, patient-centric means that you as a company work hard to meet many patients with the illness and talk to them to learn how the illness works for them, and spend time with their family, as this will often tell you a different side of the illness. Don't just send us a questionnaire, or a five-minute survey and ask us silly things like 'in the last seven days have you had trouble walking?'. This teaches you nothing, I am tempted to write yes to this question, but then add a note saying that it might have been the bottle of wine I downed rather than the illness. I wonder what a researcher would write down for the answer if they saw that response.

Find out about the impact of the illness and see if we have other illnesses alongside the one you are investigating; maybe there is a link between the illnesses that could lead to a breakthrough (and possibly even more profits for you as a company).

When I started out working at a Pharma company before university and a medical device company after university, I had the confidence and energy of youth. But I never believed I would be affected by the things I was working on or writing about; they seemed a million miles away from my own life. **The industry is full of these people: intelligent, educated, excited to succeed, ambitious and utterly blind to the impact they can have on a person's life.**

I was keen and wanted to make a real difference in my early career. I was very eager to understand and make an impact on patients' lives. So, what if we could harness all those dreams? What if, as people enter the industry and are placed within a specific therapy or illness area, they were given a chance to learn and understand the illness and those who suffer from it? A formal process of training, like the training they receive for the products. It would not take long to embed some real-world experience, not an ideal textbook patient or one selected because they fit the current focus of the company, but real patients, warts and all. Surely for the industry, this would give a well-rounded individual who can make the company genuinely patient-centric and enable it to use the power of youthful ambition in a positive manner going forward.

**Should you call me a patient?**

Another conversation I have been personally involved in (obviously before being diagnosed, as people would probably be embarrassed to have this conversation in front of me now). Should I be described as a Patient, an End-user, a Consumer or a Customer? This is a hard decision because while I receive the treatment, I believe I am a patient, but I am a patient in my relationship to the doctor or hospital, not a patient of the pharma industry. If I am not receiving treatment, even if I have a chronic illness, I do not see myself as a patient as this implies, I am ill. I can have my illness but, if it is controlled, I am not constantly sick, I am stuck in no man's land, between good health and illness.

It is quite acceptable for my doctors to call me the patient; this is the right description of our relationship. Although I am the patient in this situation, I should still have input into the decisions around my health, and I expect the respect to flow both ways between doctor and patient. We should be equal partners in our fight. I would never consider myself the patient of the medical industry, even if I am involved in a trial for them; they are not my doctor, and I am not their patient.

So, this leaves us with 'End-user', 'Consumer' or 'Customer', plus probably a few other choice words, but here is my opinion. I am the End-user of most of the drugs/devices, and I am happy with that title, but I know this doesn't sound very glamorous. But to me, this is what I am: the end of the line. The product may be sold to somebody further up the chain and the person paying for it may not be the person choosing it for my use, but I am the person who gets it and therefore hopefully gets the benefit. So, End-user is ok with me, but it is not used that much as it doesn't sound very grand.

Both Consumer and Customer stick in my throat; they make me feel like I'm off on a shopping spree like I need some glossy magazines to describe my life and choices. This is a step away from reality because, if I were an actual consumer or customer, I would choose not to need the product at all. If I look at it from a different angle, these two words imply that I have full control around the choice of my treatment, which is so far from reality, it is laughable. I don't have the clinical knowledge to make this decision on my own, and there are money and regulatory constraints, so there is just no way I can independently decide which product I will try next. So, industry, please do not patronise and pretend that I have a consumer choice about the decisions. Let's face it, if I really had an option, I would have no contact with any Pharma or medical products ever again, this isn't a choice.

**Maybe you could just call me a 'person who has xxx', as in reality, I am a person, just like you, but I happen to have a diagnosed chronic illness. The most powerful thing you can do is to treat me as a person. This works for me.**


**Patient advocates**

As patients, we may be keen to share our stories, trying to help others living with our illness, and if we are asked by hospitals, or companies to 'represent' our group of people, some of us will jump at this. I touched earlier on how the industry loves to use 'patient advocates' or 'professional patients'. These are people who have an illness and want to help others by talking about their experiences, issues and practical solutions. People go into this with the highest motivation and genuinely believe they are helping their fellow sufferers, and they really do help.

Each person is unique and faces their own individual battle, as in the rest of life; some experiences will overlap, but they will not all be the same. For me, it is like listening to a female politician when they stand up and say 'I understand all single mothers because I am a single mother. This MP is not like all other single mothers; I find it condescending that she then assumes she understands all the struggles single mothers face. It is insulting to assume that, because you have one thing in common, you can speak for a set 'segment' of the population.

To all the patients out there who have shared their stories (like I am doing now with this book), please do not take what I am saying as a personal attack. It is not; you are super brave and should continue to talk about your experiences. Stories give others strength and they push our information into newspapers and magazines. Keep going, but make sure it is your story you tell and not versions of your narrative that may be suggested to better fit the requirements of a company, journal or programme. Give your honest opinions and feedback and share facts openly.

To Industry, be careful about how you use your advocates. They are people with feelings who want to help other people. They represent some of our challenges, but to correctly understand the fight we have, you need to listen to more than one or two of the people. To publicly link with a couple of patients as your support network for knowledge and feedback does not give you the full story; this becomes a PR exercise in showing how you care. However, it does not mean you have listened; please ensure you hear the stories and really use the information you are privileged to be given. Don't just try and search out the patients who have the set criteria to support your latest product launch, instead involve patients early on in product development and talk to us about where we really need help in our daily lives.

**Remember, some people have been left so distressed by their illnesses that they remain hidden away from the world. If you can search out these patients, you will find a different reality: you will discover pain and fragility, and an honesty that will be hard to face. These are the people who really need you to be patient-centric and find**

them a cure, with urgency. They may be very different from the more confident patients who actively share their stories.

## Surveys and questionnaires

To really start to understand how you can help us live with the illness, ask us questions about our life, and how the symptoms and treatment side-effects influence our life and the choices we make. Try and understand the battles we wake up to every morning, and if you cannot cure us, then work with us to help build us a better life; ask our families about the struggles they see every day and how they deal with the battles we face.

I would love to think that there is product development out there for a new version of steroids, the wonder drug that has saved so many lives but the side-effects of which have also damaged so many of our days. To have a steroid that gives us all the benefits with none or limited side-effects would be amazing, but I don't think there is an alternative coming. Could this be because steroids are no longer under patent and are therefore sold cheaply? It would require a financial incentive to convince healthcare professionals to use new drugs with no side-effects so the drug companies would struggle to charge a high price for the new drug. Therefore the profits will never be in the 'blockbuster' range.

So, as a challenge, if any industry representative is truly 'patient-centric', find a steroid replacement without the horrendous side-effects. This would change a lot of people's lives, and for me personally, I would not be sat here writing this with my legs raised because my knees are swollen beyond recognition, causing me significant discomfort.

Surveys can be like statistics: if you are looking to show something, you will be able to find a way to manipulate the data to support your argument. For example, if you are ready to launch a new product and all your internal details are prepared, you need a few 'patient stories' or quotes, and how you go about finding them will depend on the message you want to deliver.

You will have seen some of these over the years,

- 'since using xxx I have had so much more energy, last week I was able to climb Everest',
- 'since I started on xxx my life is so much easier, I just got married to my wonderful husband, and we are off to the Bahamas'.

These stories are the best of the best.  Now, I did not climb mountains before I got ill, and I don't really want to think that because of some brilliant product I will aim to get to the top of Everest.  Sometimes, these stories really are the cream of the crop: patients who maybe had a mild strain of illness or who were very fit and healthy before the treatment or are massively driven people.  The stories are not always representative of us average patients.  Think of these stories as like the proportion of fit and healthy people who climb Everest compared to those who decide not to climb mountains ever in their lives.  It is a small percentage of people who will complete the 'ultra' challenges.  I'm not sure Hollywood will be queueing up to sign me up for the movie poster reading:

"I managed to get up today and got dressed and looked presentable on the school run." Woooohhhhooooo.

**Clinical Trials**

Clinical trials must be fair, and companies must be honest with the people taking part as they are in a moment of fragility. Illness brings many worries and stress, and any research should not add the additional unnecessary concern to patients or families. Treat people with respect, ensure trials are investigating the right things and publish ALL results, whether they were a success or failure.  A clinical trial with a negative outcome may lead to ideas or development in other areas, but if the findings are not published, then possible connections and lessons will never be found, shared or utilised.

## Working together

I am not naive, I know companies are created to make a profit, and I know that without profits the company will not survive. I know that universities need research grants, and without grants, the research will stop. I know governments are full of politicians concerned about their own careers. To cure illness, we need money coming in: we need to sell products or services to fund future research. This system (and I really don't know how we solve this) means that teams and companies and universities work in silos, often 'racing' each other to get to the solution first. The first company to market often attains substantially more profit than the company who arrives second or third. These market forces work well for say a smartphone, pushing the market for new developments and driving innovation.

Having watched this industry from the commercial side and the patient side, I think healthcare is very different from other sectors. Yes, profits are high, but investment in research is high, and there are thousands of sub-sectors of the industry. Each sub-sector is very different and cannot be really considered as the same industry. Look at a few different treatments or illnesses that you know and think about the education, knowledge and expertise the person designing the treatment must undertake. Nobody understands all the illnesses, treatments or services available worldwide, it is an enormously diverse mega-industry. Yet so many illnesses are inter-related, and people often have more than one illness that should ideally be assessed and treated together.

As patients, our GP frequently reviews our overall health and the interplay between illnesses, and generally, they are excellent at diagnosing and identifying the best ways to deal with them. Whether our best option is a pill, counselling or a referral to a clinical specialist, they are our central point of reference. However, when we go off to a specialist in the hospital, do they review our overall health or just the part they are interested in?  As a patient, you need to be the one to ensure you tell them about other areas that may interrelate.  I use the starter sentence:

'I'm not sure all these points are related but do you mind if I just run through them quickly and you can decide if they are important.'

Your GP can also help you with identifying connected symptoms, but remember you need to take the initiative to ask for help in this area.

Changes are being made to improving the visibility of clinical trials and ensuring that the data from trials are shared, even if the trial is not a success.  This is a step forward, but there is still significant work to do.

What about sharing the early stage research or anonymous patient questionnaires, or university research programs, or share when a Clinical Consultant uses a product 'off-label' (this means they use a product in a way which that the manufacturer does not have the approval to promote use in that aspect) for a different illness as they believe it will work?  This information isn't always shared in a structured manner.  If all this information were available publicly, would we see faster development, fast crossover of solutions between illness treatments?

The industry continues to work in silos trying to get the 'breakthrough product' first, which means there is a lot of money thrown at research.  I don't believe it is always done efficiently; it leads to a significant amount of duplication of early development work.  Please share all information so that we don't waste time, please work across scientific disciplines and organisations to solve some of the world's health issues.  If it is down to profits, then governments and financers you need to step in, as this is not a standard industry.  If I don't get a new smartphone for six months, it is not going to kill me; if you delay getting my treatment approved by six months, I may not survive that delay.  **It is as simple as that: delays will kill people like me.**

I was surprised when I was first diagnosed; I worked with professional experts from many different technological disciplines, and yet these lovely highly qualified and experienced people knew very little about my new illness. They knew their products and their area of the industry, but there was minimal sharing of knowledge across different product classes or illness segments.

All I could think was 'there may be a cure out there, but nobody has thought to try it on my illness'. We can see research going on for Alzheimer's patients using drugs initially designed for stroke patients[25]. These are two illnesses which have been heavily studied for many years; what if more treatments could cross over to other areas? How do we discover these opportunities? Who can think outside their current target market? How do we work together: patients, companies, researchers, money people and policymakers?

Researchers and developers, please understand not just your illness area and the symptoms, look at the patient as a complete package - view the whole picture. Look at other promising areas of research, read about other breakthroughs and consider how you could work with other disciplines of engineering, science and technology. **Some of us are desperate, and if there is a possibility of finding a solution that is already partially developed or fully available, please look for the opportunity. Think as if you are searching to cure yourself, please.**

### Healthcare workers

I have spent a long time in NHS establishments in the UK, and I have spent a long time working in companies with high customer focus and stringent expectations placed upon their employees. I observed a very different work ethos between many staff in healthcare settings, whether that be a hospital, doctors' surgeries, or care settings, and those who work in the shareholder-led industry. Please let me make clear this is a

---

[25] Association between stroke and Alzheimer's disease: systematic review and meta-analysis.

Zhou J1, Yu JT2, Wang HF3, Meng XF4, Tan CC4, Wang J4, Wang C4, Tan L2. https://www.ncbi.nlm.nih.gov/pubmed/25096624

generalisation, and there are genuinely fantastic healthcare professionals I have met along the journey.

Unfortunately, these amazing people can be let down by less conscientious colleagues. Walking into hospital wards in the UK can feel like walking into a room of people waiting to meet the tax man: not happy or positive, just dull, boring and downright miserable. Yes, I know the people are ill, and some may be waiting to meet their maker, but this does not excuse the staff from trying to ensure that their time in the hospital is a positive experience. Don't worry, I am not suggesting that the healthcare team break into an energetic dance routine with jazz hands. It is about the simple things.

**Remember you are dealing with humans, please.**

We know you are busy and stressed, but please can you remember that we are humans, and as such would prefer you not to shout our issues out loud so that everybody can hear? Why don't you ask us questions about 'why we are here' instead of searching the computer screen for ten minutes trying to find the start of our problems? Most of us can still talk and are awake enough to give you a quick summary. We are people; why don't you look at us when you talk to us? I lay on my bed once and watched three doctors speak to a computer screen, asking each other when I was first diagnosed. Eventually, I interrupted them and told them the date; they looked surprised... maybe they thought I couldn't speak?

Another big issue for me is privacy and respect. I don't allow anybody to grab me without asking, 'do would you mind if I just...'? Just because I am in a hospital bed does not mean I have lost all my personality or inhibitions; I am quite shy about my body and think it would be nice if you, a) told me what you plan to do and then, b) asked if it was ok to do it.

Wards are the most inhumane and depressing places you can find; it is tough to keep your dignity and hygiene when there are eight of you sharing a bathroom. I always try to get up, get dressed and face the world, but some days it is not possible, and I would like some help. But it really is not necessary to talk to me like a child and manhandle me like you are playing with a doll that you hate (or possibly a voodoo doll that if you inflict pain on me, it is transferred to somebody you do not like); please handle me with care.

Maybe just treat us as you would like to be treated, regardless of our age, sex, nationality, language, religion or illness; surely, we all deserve that amount of respect?

Can you also remember that, although this is your day job and you are used to the routines, details and sometimes extreme treatment, it is likely to be the first time that we have faced this? Please understand our fear and help us to deal with the situation. **We don't know what is happening or what any of it means. Use simple words and explain things, be friendly and help us to relax. No matter what we say or how we act, we are scared and unsure of what will happen to us next.**

**You are the examples that we look to, whether you like that idea or not.**

As a healthcare professional, we know you went through training for many years, and that you understand the damage that massive bag of crisps can do to the body. And yet, sometimes when we look at you, it is difficult to be encouraged by your words if your own personal actions do not back up the advice you are giving us patients.

A proportion of ward healthcare staff appears from the outside to be incredibly miserable, unhealthy and sometimes overweight. Patients sit in their beds and listen to you giving us advice on a healthier lifestyle and how to prevent illnesses, but often your words do not match the expression on your face. The words then become empty, and it is hard for us to 'buy into' your message. If you want me to lose two stone, as this will drastically decrease the chance of the illness flaring, can you understand my scepticism of your words when I look, and you must be at least a stone heavier than me? It is not inspiring. I am sorry if this sounds horrible; it is horrible, I am saying a horrible thing, but this is the reality of the thoughts going through your patients' minds.

If you can smile your patients will more than likely smile back at you, and then smile at other patients and who knows, within an hour, the whole ward may have a gentle little smile. Maybe the same with healthy eating and positivity. It would be so much better for the patients to spend the whole day in a ward of people who are not miserable in their job and how great would it be for you to come into work and have your patients smile at you.

**You can escape each night, we cannot.**

When you go home at night, you can take your shoes off, sit quietly with a cup of tea, or relax in a bath, while we patients are stuck in the hospital, sharing a bathroom with strangers, eating cold food and only getting hot drinks when we are told we can have them. It is lonely, scary and totally lacking in privacy. We conform to your routine, you wake us up at 6 am for tests, give us nightly injections, even when we are not sure why we need them. The lack of privacy was my biggest issue; I found it very difficult to be around strangers for 24-hours a day with everybody watching, constantly. To me, hospital feels like a prison where my freedom has been taken away, a prison I know I need to stay in, but that feels like a horrible place to be.

It is not just the prison feeling, but also the fact that the reality of being ill is forced on you. As you will know by now, I work extremely hard to act like I am not ill. Hospital's remove this luxury, with discussions on how you feel every few hours, a nurse who gives you your tablets that you usually take on your own at home but are not allowed to in the hospital. It is all a constant reminder that you really are quite ill. The no flowers rule leave the wards a very 'dry' place to be. I was very grateful during my last stay when I got the bed by the window, because:

1. I only had another patient to one side of me, so when I wanted some quiet time, I could turn to the side where I was not looking at anybody and have

a little bit of privacy. People still talk to you, but you can at least pretend not to be there for a short space of time or pretend to be asleep.

2. I could see a small shed at the end of the hospital grounds; it must have only been a little 'sentinel' shed, maybe a metre square. But I dreamt of what was in that shed, about who went and hid inside its secret walls. I never saw anybody go in or out, but I watched the small flowers around the shed and dreamt of being out in the countryside and smelling the flowers. It was a window which allowed me to escape the facts of the internal hospital ward.

During all my stays in hospitals, I have been in wards which generally have people older than me in them, who have always been amazingly realistic and funny. They have looked at the world from a different perspective than me. One astonishing 84-year-old who was seriously ill told me that she prayed to God for me. When I said that I would do the same, she asked why; she said she had had her fun, seen her children grow up and get married, laughed, cried and been very naughty, but that now it was her time to make way for others. I was left speechless.

These lovely ladies took an interest in others that is not seen in the world outside life on the ward, and at first, I found the questions, conversations and rather loud comments about me, to their family as a problem. But over time, I realised that they were reassuring, kind and genuine; the ward becomes a community, that like any community has its positives and negatives. The positives are that you share the experience and support each other. You try and entertain your community and ensure they are looked after properly (like when at 3am one of them rolled out of bed on the opposite side to the drip stand that she was connected too. I am not sure I have ever moved so fast out of my bed). The negatives are that there is always noise, always something happening, always somebody listening and commenting. Even when you hear the bad news, you must face your community, knowing they have listened to the same information. It is really very hard to deal with all of this, but I am not sure I would change it for the world because sometimes, just sometimes, it is just what you need.

My bed by the window took on extra importance when, on day three of my stay, the worst happened. A lady had been brought in for a routine operation but had developed a severe infection, which meant she didn't regain any meaningful consciousness. In respect to her, I won't give many details. For days her family visited, and we heard all the conversations with the doctors.

**DOCTORS, PLEASE NOTE, A CURTAIN DOES NOT BLOCK SOUND – WE CAN HEAR EVERYTHING.**

Then one evening about 11.30pm she breathed for the last time.

I cannot explain the sadness I felt for this stranger who I had never spoken too, but I felt such a deep connection with her in her last moments. I cried silently under the covers. Then I realised the other five people in the room were awake and crying; we looked at each other, not sure what to do. The staff called the doctor, who pronounced the time of death, and then they left her body there, all night. Her family came and cried and shouted and cried. And we all lay in our beds trying to pretend we couldn't hear through that bloody curtain. We comforted each other, we cuddled, and we each checked we were all ok.

No staff member said anything to us or checked how we were. We stayed in the ward with her body until the morning.

This is no way to die, and this is no way to be treated when you die; surely, there is a way to give the respect that should be there in these circumstances. Death occurs in hospitals, I understand that, and I appreciate that healthcare professionals may be used to dealing with it. But fellow patients are not, and it scares us even more than we were before; it makes us fearful that we may follow and then be treated in the same unemotional manner. Please remember that this may be our first-time seeing death, it was mine.

# Your first job is to care

**Please, please, please care for us. Don't see us as an inconvenience: we don't want to be there, and we don't want to cause you issues. But we need to be there, and we need your help and care. Treatment is essential to us, but feeling cared for while we face all this is more important.** Throughout all the miracle drugs and tests we are scared, we are in a strange place with total strangers... while dressed in our pyjamas! Over the years, I have met some astonishing healthcare workers who genuinely care beyond the requirements of their career. I am so grateful to every one of you, thank you. I have also met many who didn't show an ounce of compassion or concern, people who made me feel like an inconvenience, which makes a difficult situation harder. I understand that some days we don't always feel like smiling; I am not talking about this. I am talking about negatively discussing patients very loudly; shouting at the old lady while giving her a bed bath; or moaning when the lady fell out of bed because you just made a hot drink and now it will go cold while you check her over. I am not suggesting you need to be a faultless saint, but if patients annoy you that much, maybe you should be in another career away from the caring professions.

Doctors, you are not excluded from this. Please, can you bring back some old-fashioned bed-side manners?

One of the best doctors I have spoken with was a military doctor working in a mainstream hospital; I had a chest infection which two lots of antibiotics had not helped, and I was admitted for IV antibiotics. I felt dreadful and really was scared. A nurse had made me concerned as she was telling me that I couldn't have a chest infection as I didn't have a temperature, and she wasn't sure why they were treating me. Not the most caring of comments.

I had seen many doctors over the preceding years, but this one doctor came to my bedside while I was physically upset with the situation. He sat on the bed and talked to me, explaining that the steroids and immune suppression drugs can prevent me from showing any signs of the immune system working, including having a temperature. It took ten minutes, and it all made sense; I thanked him, and he smiled. I will NEVER forget that conversation. In fact, I often repeat some of the comments he shared if I am seeing a doctor I have not seen before, just to point out that I am a little special.

That small kindness, talking to me like a human, made a tremendous positive impact on me and my life. Other experiences have been where doctors speak over my head like I am not there, and I don't remember what they said or who they were. **If you want patients to listen and understand, talk to them with care and honesty, and generally how you would want others to speak to you if the roles were reversed.**

## Tell us the truth

**Don't tell me a treatment will work if, realistically, the chance of improving my situation is only about 20%. Give me the facts and let my family and I make informed decisions.** I am quite clear that I do not want to receive two months of horrible treatment that will leave me in a terrible state if it will only prolong my life by a couple of months. Give me the time so I can go outside, see the sun and enjoy my days. Don't leave me hooked up to a machine.

Please don't do things for the sake of it. Think about whether you would choose to have the treatment, or whether you would allow your children to go down that route, if you wouldn't, and then tell us about your reservations, explain the positive and negatives and let us decide. But our decision should be made after hearing the complete facts. I hope that when I reach the last few months of life, whether I am 105 or 60 years old, I can die with dignity in the manner I choose. I am sure the preferred choice will not be hooked up to a machine and leaving the world in the presence of a room full of strangers. I choose a shorter life, but one with dignity, with family and friends around me.

I understand that we need innovation, and I am desperate for some amazing invention to help my situation. But just because you have a shiny new machine or medicine, don't feel that you must use it on me.  Are you sure it will help?  If not, then give me the full facts and let me decide on the risks.  Would you use it on yourself?  We need treatments to be safe and effective, and I really don't mind if that means using something that has been around for 40 years.

**Charities**

Charities do keep going, you are there to support people and push for effective treatment; this is about raising money. Please do not scare people into donating or badger them.  Make sure your team are aware of the limitations that they should not cross.  Charities are there to fight for good, and we understand that you must run as a business and meet all the regulatory requirements; do not cross the lines and become solely about getting money, no matter how you do this.

Work together with other charities, there are advantages to sharing information. There are often several charities for an illness or a group of patients.  It would be good to work together and pool your knowledge and funds so that you become more effective.  You may have complementary research which leads to a breakthrough when you combine your understanding.  Do not to compete; what is the value in this?

Many charities startup in memory of a person, which is impressive and I do not know where people get the strength to do this.  Running a charity is hard work; it is the equivalent of running a business, and often it may not run for a very long time because of the stress and continuous effort needed.  Could your passions be used more effectively if you joined an established charity and built some events in honour of your lost one, so the money and support go to the established charity with the infrastructure and funds to drive for real change?  I understand this is not the same for remembering the person, but in the longer term it may lead to the change you are fighting for; you could join the charity's board of directors or support them in another way.

When we get ill, we need people to trust, and we need information we can believe. We may need somebody to talk to or somebody who can understand us. The charity I have leaned on has been fantastic; it is run by volunteers, and they are amazingly supportive. I am in awe of the energy and love they give, totally selflessly and never-ending. X.

Please stay ethical and remember why you were created; stay true to your mission.

**Governments**

Governments, please see the health industry as different from other sectors; don't make it all about money. I hear lots of comments about the money going into the NHS and how we need more and more and more. I disagree with this, the NHS could work smarter and more efficient, like any big organisation, but throwing endless buckets of money at this will not help patients. You need to work with our health services and listen: listen to the healthcare professionals, the patients and the charities. Then learn, from what you hear, from best practice in business, from efficiencies gained from technology. Motivate your teams, motivate patients to be proactive, and build a strong network of passionate people willing to fight to make the service the best it can be. There are so many people out there who want to devote their lives to making healthcare work, don't exasperate these people, please.

The lack of trust between the NHS and the UK government is terrifying. The NHS is one of the most amazing ideas on the planet: free healthcare when you need it. But to provide this, the systems in the background must be set up correctly, the staff must be motivated and believe in their management. IT systems are often antiquated, staff unmotivated, and there is a huge gap between management and frontline staff... and I know this from sitting in a hospital waiting rooms, wards and hospital restaurants listening. No surveys needed, the comments are freely said out loud. There is a general misery amongst NHS staff that no amount of money will solve. I don't have the answers, but I know that when a workforce is as unhappy as this, then somebody is not listening.

Politicians, please don't destroy one of the wonders of the world to protect your political career.

One of my other messages to governments is around charities. I understand that you cannot fund all the research needed, but please can you monitor the activities of charities and the destination of the funds? Not all charities are looking after the interests of patients; it is your role to monitor this with the charities commission and act if needed. Charities are taking money from emotional and often vulnerable people, who may not be thinking rationally; you need to protect these people.

Many illnesses have outstanding and successful charities supporting them, but a lot do not. Surely you must take some responsibility for these people and help them when there is nobody else to support them. When I had chemotherapy, I really wanted some support for my daughter, somebody for her to talk to who understood, but because I didn't have cancer, there were no support groups available to offer help. Surely this is not right. She needed help but couldn't get any, even though her needs were arguably the same as the child whose parent has cancer. Can you help in this situation? Support like this should not really depend on the type of illness a person has to live with or how much money a charity can generate. It is not fair that patients suffer because there isn't a big charity to support them.

You make the laws of our land; you can make significant changes if you wanted. Why not start with some simple changes? Only ethically approve trials where the companies will share research and real information with the general public, and do not allow them to hide negative results.

Be strict on rogue companies or charities, these companies can cause death by their actions. Get experts in this area and drive legislation that pushes the healthcare industries to be the most efficient and ethical in the world.

Incentivise companies to work together and really have patients at the centre of their focus, rather than profits. You have this power, why do you not use it? Instead, you argue about a few million more investment into the NHS, which, if we are honest, will make no difference to the overall service.

You can motivate healthcare staff, support them, engage with them, and protect them from stupid legal cases which make some of them too scared to practice. Fight for these teams; if you fight and treasure them, you will see a more significant benefit than throwing money and hoping and praying for a solution. Talk to professionals, talk to patients, borrow expertise from other industries and other countries… seek to improve and drive progress for all our benefits.

In a nutshell: Please go to work every day like it is your life you are working towards saving. One day your efforts may change your own life, and how happy will you be to have fully committed to your job in the past.

## Changes we can make from today; master of my fate.

The changes we can make going forward depend very much on our past journey, our illness, our support network, our treatment and our planned future. I cannot tell you what you need to do, I will just explain how I expect to face every new day.

1. First, I will remember the Invictus poem and realise that my battle can be partly in my brain: the battle to stay positive and live with the life I have today, to get up and get the most out of the day. Life may never be the same as pre-diagnosis, but that does not mean it cannot still be fun and full of adventure (even if sometimes I need extra help or a quick afternoon sleep).

2. I will take responsibility for my treatment: I will read, I will do my research and push for the right things for me. I will respect the NHS but also understand the immense pressure placed on it, so I will do my part to support the NHS in treating me. I will become knowledgeable about my condition and try to understand my symptoms and identify when I need to go and seek medical help.

3. I will follow my treatment plans and the instructions I am given from the experts. However, if I doubt the regime, I will question the expert who has prescribed the plan. If, when I have asked my questions, I am still not satisfied, I will search out answers that do make sense, and if necessary, seek a second opinion.

4. I will spend time with friends and family and make the most of relationships with those I love.

5. I WILL NOT Google for advice but will use trusted websites (see the end of the book). If I cannot find a reliable site, I will ask my doctor or patient association representative for recommendations. (Also, personally, I will never read health advice from the UK newspapers).

6. If possible, I will actively take part in research, and push to see the results of any investigation. I will also have a quick search of alltrials.com to see what is relevant to me.

7. I will (try) not to feel sorry for myself, or ask 'why me?' I will (try to) accept that my condition is now part of my life and find a way to continue to live it to the maximum. When I fail at this one, I will not be hard on myself, just start the next day afresh.

8. I will make sure I look after myself by eating well and making sure I get moving, no matter how slowly, every day.

9. I won't waste money on miracle cures that do not have any evidence in science.

10. I will keep fighting to do these things every day, as I must not give in to this illness when there is still so much fun to be had!

## Final word

By the way, you have reached the end of the book and not once have I told you what illness I have been given as a gift. This was on purpose; the specific illness doesn't matter for many of the things I have written about. Many of the coping techniques for chronic illnesses centre around our brain and our determination, not our physical hindrance. For those interested, I have two types of rare autoimmune Vasculitis (with a knackered thyroid and asthma thrown in). It isn't nice, but I will not lie down and give in; Pac man you are not catching me today.

Keep your spirit, keep your fight, rest, don't be hard on yourself and smile.

Remember the Invictus words:

**I am the master of my fate:**
**I am the captain of my soul.**

# Reference website

**UK**

- NHS Choices: **www.nhs.UK**
- UK clinical Trails gateway: **www.ukctg.nihr.ac.uk/**
- MHRA (UK regulatory authority) Yellow card reporting system, for unexpected incidents with treatment: **https://yellowcard.mhra.gov.uk/**
- NICE UK Government department: **www.nice.org.uk/**
- Patient Social Media site: **healthunlocked.com/**
- UK Rare Illness support: **www.rareillness.org.uk/**

**Europe**

- EU news on healthcare issues: **ec.europa.eu/health/home_en**
- Rare illness: **www.eurordis.org/**
- Patient Association: **www.eu-patient.eu/**

**North America**

- FDA **https://www.fda.gov/patients**
- US National Cancer Institute: **www.cancer.gov/**
- Mayo Clinic **www.mayoclinic.org/patient-care-and-health-information**
- Cleveland Clinic; **my.clevelandclinic.org/health**

If you want more details:

- **www.testingtreatments.org/** free electronic version of the book, plus resources about treatment claims, the content is available in many languages.

- **www.cochrane.org** Cochrane is a global independent network of researchers, professionals, patients, carers and people interested in health.

- **www.ncbi.nlm.nih.gov/pubmed** PubMed comprises more than 28 million citations for biomedical literature from MEDLINE, life science journals, and online books. Citations may include links to full-text content from PubMed Central and publisher websites.

- World Health Organisation: **http://apps.who.int/trialsearch/**

If you do need to search google, go through Google Scholar.

## About the Author: Jane L Edwards

I am a mother of two, living in Lincolnshire, who still has her ambitions, but I am now physically hindered from meeting some of these dreams. It has been a very long journey to complete this book, and I really hope that it can offer some support to you.

My world revolves around my family and my wonderful Labrador who have all helped me through the battles.

This is my first book and is an extremely personal story to tell.

Quick legal comment, this book is my journey, none of the statements is personal advice for you, if you need personalised help, please speak with your doctor.

Copyright @2019 Jane L Edwards

ISBN 9781075727863

All rights reserved.

Printed in Great Britain
by Amazon